LOOKING BACK

TO LOOK
FORWARD

LOOKING BACK

TO LOOK FORWARD

AUPHA AT 70

Michael R. Meacham, JD, Editor

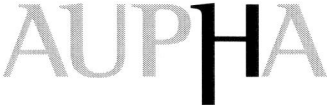

Association of University Programs in Health Administration
Washington, DC

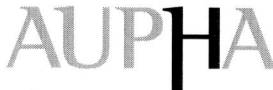

In the evolution of any major organization, especially one that has survived 70 years, it is natural to recognize the influential presidents, chairs, and award winners as we have done in this book. We also identified the many members who wrote articles for the book, contributed side perspectives on the articles, and contributed to the book's "construction." It would be remiss, however, not to recognize the many others, many now deceased, who provided the fuel for AUPHA. Faculty leaders who worked without guidelines or recognition outside of their university to develop, nurture, and sustain their programs as the field grew. These individuals were loyal members of AUPHA for over 70 years. Countless other faculty and staff who may not have attained senior leadership roles in their programs or in AUPHA but nonetheless contributed through service on committees and task forces at the behest of AUPHA leaders. Many other faculty attended and contributed to the richness of such activities as our meetings, faculty forums, webinars, and journal articles. Finally, the overlapping members who attended or participated in the meetings of our affiliated professional organizations at the local, regional, and national levels. This effort supported AUPHA's crucial connection to the American College of Healthcare Executives, American Hospital Association, Medical Group Management Association, Healthcare Information and Management Systems Society, Healthcare Financial Management Association, Academy of Management, AcademyHealth, and many other organizations. These often unnamed individuals contributed greatly to AUPHA without the benefit of significant visibility, and certainly without pay! This book is dedicated to you all, those who made AUPHA what it is today.

Contents

Preface

Gary L. Filerman, PhD

THE ASSOCIATION OF University Programs in Health Administration (AUPHA) was created in 1948 as a component of a carefully thought-out and crafted social intervention. The objective of the W.K. Kellogg Foundation was to improve the performance of hospitals. A central strategy was to build the professionalism and competencies of their administrators. It was an extraordinarily successful demonstration of the ability of a private foundation to bring change by focusing resources and leadership on a problem that affected the quality of life.

The need for action following World War II had been recognized by Kellogg and a couple of other foundations by supporting graduate programs in hospital administration. These were fragile experimental ventures, dependent on the leadership of a few individuals who had status in hospital administration practice but who mostly lacked academic credentials; the programs had small, mainly part-time faculties and were situated in schools that were less than enthusiastic supporters. It was to the programs' advantage that the initiative coincided with the period when universities were confronting the need to integrate problem-centered education with discipline-based organizations.

When the program leaders formed their association, they drew on their experiences as participants in professional organizations. The objective was to have a place for collegial interaction and shared experience, and to provide a base for program representation and recognition by the two dominant hospital organizations, the American College of Hospital Administrators (later American College of Healthcare Executives) and the American Hospital Association. They gradually added academic development activities and even a process for setting and applying standards for membership in the club.

As the investor in most of the programs, Kellogg, in the person of Andrew Pattullo, was an interested participant observer of these activities. After about 15 years, he felt that the point had been made. The programs had survived and grown, new programs were attracting good students, the ranks of academically qualified faculty were increasing, and the graduates were getting the intended jobs. He concluded that the return on investment should be considerably greater. However, what had not developed was a vison of how the programs, through the association, should and could make a more consequential contribution to the growth of the academic enterprise and to the performance of the delivery system. Obliquely, he invited a proposal for a more ambitious agenda. All that follows in this story flows from that decision and the support that followed.

The agenda had two objectives: strengthen the core curricula and provide the organizational capacity to support that effort. Many faculty members were involved in the development of the programmatic response to the opportunity, which generated a vision and the organizing concept that was to define the culture of AUPHA for at least the next 30 years.

AUPHA was defined as an academic consortium, owned by and for the programs and their faculties. The mission was to provide leadership through a collegial platform that responded to the needs and interests of the programs and faculties. It was to foster program and faculty growth by creative opportunism. It was to be distinctly different from the trade associations of other health professions programs and schools.

Organizations are organisms that evolve in response to changing leadership, their environment, opportunities, constituents, competition, and resources. I suggest that these are appropriate lenses through which to view the evolution of AUPHA from its youth to middle age. The six strategic objectives that emerged in the first decade and determined the association's programmatic priorities were the following:

1. Promote the visibility and stature of the programs and the faculties on the campus and in the broader academic, professional, and donor communities. Gain a seat for the profession at relevant policy tables.
2. Provide opportunities for faculty members from many disciplines to contribute to and to benefit from participation. Build broad faculty ownership beyond program directors.
3. Establish an academic infrastructure to include a recognized accreditation program to achieve eligibility for federal support, establish a peer-reviewed journal to stimulate education research, and expand teaching resources and publishing opportunities by establishing a publishing venture.
4. Support faculty participation in health services research.
5. Develop a recruitment program to expand the pool of high-potential students. Expand diversity in the field.
6. Enhance employer and practitioner recognition of the value added to the field by the graduates and the programs.

These priorities, refined and implemented in the early years, provide benchmarks against which to view the organization's subsequent development. As I assess their sustainability, clearly a persistent challenge has been how to capitalize on the strength of AUPHA's unique mix of program settings and faculty disciplines. All things considered, it has done quite well.

All that AUPHA has accomplished and will accomplish is the result of the commitment to the mission by many faculty members and the staff. In the context of this history, it is important to note the extraordinary interest, support, time, and energy contributed in the beginning by visionary leaders in the field: Andrew Pattullo (W.K. Kellogg Foundation), George Bugbee (University of Chicago), Ray E. Brown (University of Chicago and Duke University), and John D. Thompson (Yale University). They were companions on the journey.

Asked to describe the orchestra, legendary composer and conductor Ernst von Dohnányi replied, "A great orchestra is greater than the sum of each member bringing his brick." AUPHA's story is the history of hundreds of faculty members and friends bringing their bricks.

As inscribed on the entrance to
the National Archives of the United States:

"What Is Past Is Prologue"

Acknowledgments

Michael R. Meacham, JD

WORKING ON THIS project has been both educational and rewarding. I have had the privilege of collaborating with a number of bright, dedicated people who have made this chronicle of the 70th year history of AUPHA possible.

Diane Howard, past AUPHA Board Chair, has been a stalwart in getting this project completed. Not only was this her idea, but she was the driving force behind it. She coauthored one chapter and served as both a formal and informal reviewer for several others. She also managed to keep the peace when some of the "creative tension" became more about the intensity and less about creativity. Diane's omnipresence of serenity and peace were essential in bringing this project to completion.

Likewise, current AUPHA Board Chair Keith Benson and Chair-Elect Mark Diana provided wise counsel and insight into a number of issues raised here. The edges in parts of this would be considerably "rougher" had it not been for their sagacious commentary from time to time.

Gerald Glandon and the AUPHA staff were of enormous support, particularly in preparing the appendices, making a treasure trove of documents available, and providing insight into many of the historical developments that provide the foundation for how AUPHA does its business today. We are all well served by the professionalism and commitment to the profession that is embodied in our staff.

The other true heroes are, of course, the authors. Although there are notes in each chapter describing the individuals, I would be remiss if I did not add a note of personal gratitude for all the time, energy, and talent they devoted to this project: Bill Aaronson, Leigh Cellucci, Rupert Evans, Sherril Gelmon, Jerry Glandon, Ray Grady, Diane Howard, Anthony Kovner, Peggy Leatt, Stephen Loebs, Brian Malec, Janet Porter, Bernardo Ramirez, Margaret Schulte, Lee Seidel, Dean Smith, Mary Stefl, and Dan West. This project would not have been possible without them and their enthusiastic engagement. Likewise, Brooke Hollis and Anthony Stanowski contributed very important sidebar material.

And, of course, no academic enterprise involving publishing would be complete without peer review. To the reviewers, thank you: Keith Benson, Mark Diana, Gary Filerman, Sherril Gelmon, Dan Gentry, Jerry Glandon, Diane Howard, Christy Harris Lemak, John Seavey, and Karen Wager.

The authors interviewed dozens of people for this project. Any attempt to list them all would be futile for the certainty of inadvertently omitting someone. There are several, however, who gave substantial time to helping many of us understand more about various aspects of the past. Gary Filerman, whose vast knowledge of AUPHA is without peer, helped many of the authors develop a depth of knowledge that added to the richness of their writing. His is a truly unique contribution reflecting his many years of service.

Lydia Middleton (Reed) provided a foundational background for many of the finer points included in these pages, also reflecting her near decade-long tenure as AUPHA President and CEO. Sherril Gelmon was kind enough to review several chapters in addition to coauthoring one.

Certainly, any publishing project like this requires some additional expertise that we do not have. To that end, we are grateful for our friends at Health Administration Press, Drew Baumann, Michael Cunningham, and Janet Davis, for their ability to put the finishing touches on the project and help us guide it across the finish line.

Finally, but certainly not least, is my appreciation for our editor, Kathleen Vega, whose keen eye, sharp pen, and wise counsel improved every page of this book. She is a joy to have as a colleague whose wisdom (and sense of humor) made this project the best it could be. We all owe her a debt of gratitude for her patience, professionalism, and expertise.

Introduction

Michael R. Meacham, JD

As readers embark on the pages that follow, they will find the stories of how and why the Association of University Programs in Health Administration (AUPHA) evolved, following the trajectory of growth in the profession of educating health services administrators. This volume is an engaging discussion of the "professionalization" of health services administration as the U.S. healthcare system became larger, more complex, and increasingly reliant on a variety of clinical and nonclinical specialists. Importantly, these stories are not merely regurgitations of events, but fascinating tales of and by some of the people who shaped our beloved AUPHA.

THE BIRTH OF A DISCIPLINE

The recognition that health services organizations might be better served with professionally trained administrators dates back to the first half of the 20th century (Levey & Hilsenrath, 1998). Physician objections in those days—that nonclinical administrators would be little more than resource-hoarding hoteliers—are often echoed today in differing perspectives between administrators and clinicians (Levey & Hilsenrath, 1998).

Over time, however, the need for a professional class of administrator became more apparent, and the profession became more widely accepted. Indeed, during the halcyon post–World War II era, federal funds and foundation largesse flowed freely. The federal government expanded healthcare in all respects: increased science (National Institutes of Health), increased funding for hospital construction (the Hill–Burton Act), and increased access to care (Medicare and Medicaid). Concomitantly, as the market for professionally trained health services managers expanded, so too did the number of programs within institutions of higher learning. Incidental to these ascendancies, both the federal government and foundations—most notably the W.K. Kellogg Foundation—funded a variety of studies, reports, and initiatives to expand the availability of "professionally trained management" in healthcare organizations. Thus, the small number—fewer than a dozen—of graduate programs in health services administration programs extant in the days before World War II grew, some would say in generational waves, in the postwar era (Loebs, 2001). Indeed, as the number of graduate programs in health services administration flourished, the concepts of managing healthcare enterprises percolated to the undergraduate level. This history recalls the dynamics of the expansion of the healthcare system and further describes how AUPHA itself evolved to expand beyond the exclusionary influences of graduate education to include baccalaureate-trained professionals.

As the education of healthcare services managers expanded, the hybrid nature of the profession became more confounding to university leaders. The underlying orientation—business and quasi-social services combined—was (and is) unique to healthcare. The collection of organizations embodying those oft-conflicting priorities dedicated to multiple morbidities afflicting human beings, is a subset of one. The central purpose of hospitals was not to generate a profit and increase value to owners like other service or manufacturing enterprises. Moreover, the charitably natured roots from which these organizations grew empowered a not-for-profit, community-focused ethos that has permeated the history of healthcare (Starr, 1982). Conversely, however, healthcare as a commodity requires that such organizations possess quantitative decision-making capability based on business values of profit, market share, return on investment, and other tools capable of expressing financial value. This provides the foundation for the debate about the root source of the best preparation for healthcare administrators and, thus, the preferred academic home of such programs. This debate is ultimately an adjunct of the fundamental philosophical question: Is healthcare a basic human right to which all are entitled, or is it a commodity to be available through market mechanisms? Healthcare is not a traditional business, so the fixation of profit in a business-only approach seems self-serving. On the contrary, healthcare in the United States is not a birthright; thus it is not exclusively a social service enterprise either, meaning that it needs to generate revenue to meet its costs. As has oft been repeated: "No margin, no mission." Thus, today we find healthcare services management programs in schools of allied health, business administration, public health, and even a handful within schools of medicine and nursing. Our common culture is a polyglot of philosophies emanating from the fundamental missions of these varied settings.

The debate about academic location *seems* partly settled now, however, with no clear consensus about what works "best." Slightly more than half of AUPHA-member programs are located in colleges of public health, health sciences, or allied health. Tracking program graduates and preferences of managers in the profession tells a slightly different story, however. The largest-growing segment of new members in the American College of Healthcare Executives (ACHE) comprises graduates from business school programs (Hilsenrath, 2012). While many, perhaps most, programs in health management education have settled into various colleges of allied health and/or health sciences, there is evidence of a strong preference for MBAs among healthcare executives (Broom & Hilsenrath, 2015). In the end, the field remains divided on the subject, as 50 percent of employed hospital executives have MHAs and are said to have better interpersonal skills than their MBA counterparts (Howard & Silverstein, 2011).

THE RISE OF PEER REVIEW

Similar to advances in medicine—with practitioners morphing from snake oil charlatans to science-based caregivers—training for hospital administrators has advanced over time. As health services administration graduate programs grew in number, so too did the need for assurance of quality in those programs. Thus was born the idea of peer review of graduate programs in the name of accreditation. Similarly, when undergraduate programs came into the fold, expanding the concept of peer review took the form of program certification. The profession moved to higher ground with the advent of professional standards by which to assess its educational foundation. AUPHA's catalytic role in this development is an important chapter in our collective history.

THE QUEST FOR DIVERSITY

The growth of professional healthcare administration and the evolution of its educational foundations occurred amid the magnification of society's larger social questions. A little-known fact that Medicare became leverage for integrating hospitals (mainly in the South, but wherever segregated wards existed) was an element in the larger civil rights movement (Chapin, 2015). Thus, not only was care delivery expanded, but the setting in which it was delivered (in some parts of the country) was also significantly changed, prompting changes in who delivered care and managed its resources. Progress in this struggle has been slow, evidenced by small gains over time. Nonetheless, AUPHA's leading role in the continuing transformation toward social equality is documented here. It is axiomatic to assert education is at the core of a free society that values the contributions of all races, creeds, and genders. AUPHA-member programs, in addition to evolving *with* the profession of healthcare administration, have advanced the causes of equality and inclusiveness reflected in our larger society to change the profession as well.

THE ROLE OF WOMEN IN AUPHA

The story of women in leadership of AUPHA is particularly intriguing, noting that the early days of hospital administration were dominated by nurses who assumed administrative duties. This seems consistent with the early view of clinicians that "since administration was unimportant, consign the function to a (female) nurse." Later, as the profession was gaining greater acceptance, early health administration programs created the climate for the profession to be "masculinized" by restricting the number of women admitted to graduate health administration programs. Over time, the winds of change eroded the "good old boys' club," and AUPHA came to accept women in increasing numbers, taking a leadership role vis-à-vis the industry in elevating the prominence of women.

REACHING BEYOND OUR BORDERS

This volume also recounts AUPHA's central role in expanding professionalism in health services administration to other countries. While the multifaceted expansion of healthcare in the United States motivated development of a professional class of administrators, our colleagues increasingly realized that other countries faced similar challenges that could benefit from these same administrators. They also recognized we might learn some new techniques and concepts from those we engage globally. As a result, AUPHA has long had a robust portfolio of active global initiatives detailed on these pages. AUPHA member programs have been particularly active in developing partnerships across Western Europe, Eastern Europe, and South America.

COMMUNICATING BEST PRACTICE

Of course, being a collection of educators requires that we have a mechanism for sharing "best practices," which gave rise to our *Journal of Health Administration Education (JHAE)*. AUPHA has an extensive and multifaceted history of sharing teaching techniques and research findings within the collegial family. The journal and our long-standing partnership with Health Administration Press provide evidence of AUPHA's leadership in advancing the science and pedagogy of developing management and leadership competencies among our students and in the profession.

EMBRACING TECHNOLOGY

The increasingly complex nature of healthcare administration required advancing the use of information technology in multiple forms. The number of payment sources grew, the number and types of services provided exploded, and the number of patients increased. This was the confluence from which healthcare information technology (IT) would develop. Business and clinical technologies became increasingly sophisticated, requiring IT managers to become more adroit in managing these new, complicated resources. The role of IT officer became a growing subset within health services administration. AUPHA member programs again responded to the increased demand and led in the development of specialized training for this growing cadre of health services administrators.

GROUNDING THEORY WITH EVIDENCE

In keeping with its mission of "fostering excellence and innovation in health management," AUPHA has played a supporting role in the advancement of evidence-based management. This is an important counterpart to the "evidence-based practice" gaining greater prominence among clinicians. This development has taken hold in several individual programs and is proliferating across the healthcare landscape. No doubt influenced by the demanding twins of transparency and accountability, this scientific approach to management will strengthen the professional stature of administrators and those who shape them.

MOVING FORWARD

Finally, this volume examines in detail AUPHA today. The last chapter includes data about growth in AUPHA's number of programs; major initiatives and projects; its strategic plan; and its vision for the future. Understanding that "past is prologue," this chapter opens the door to the future by examining where we have been: advanc-ing our vision through the development of leaders who will manage and lead all of us to a better healthcare system.

The pages of this volume recount for the reader a unique and complex story: the growth and development of an organization of men and women dedicated to improving the lives of humanity through the education of those who lead the development and implementation of healthcare services. It is a noble calling that has not only endured, but also thrived in its metamorphoses from its beginning at the 1948 meeting of several program directors in Roosevelt Hospital in New York City to an organization serving as the national foundation for educating highly competent professional administrators in healthcare services delivery.

REFERENCES

Broom, K., & Hilsenrath, P. (2015). ACHE member survey: Perspectives on graduate health managment education. *Journal of Health Education Administration, 32*(3), 341–358.

Chapin, C. (2015). *Ensuring America's health: The public creation of the corporate health care system.* New York, NY: Cambridge University Press.

Hilsenrath, P. (2012). Healthcare education management in the United States: History and perspective. *Journal of Management History, 18*(4), 386–401.

Howard, D. M., & Silverstein, D. (2011). *The interpersonal skills of recent entrants to the field of healthcare management: Final report.* Chicago, IL: American College of Healthcare Executives.

Levey, S., & Hilsenrath, H. J. (1998). Dilemmas in health education management: Past, present and future. *Journal of Health Administration Education, 16*(1), 61–85.

Loebs, S. (2001). The continuing evolution of health management education. *Journal of Health Administration Education,* Supplemental Issue, 33–50.

Starr, P. (1982). *The social transformation of American medicine.* New York, NY: Basic Books.

CHAPTER 1

The Profession and AUPHA: The Beginning

Michael R. Meacham, JD

INTRODUCTION

In December 1948, 15 people—11 men and 4 women—gathered at Roosevelt Hospital in New York City to take the initial steps in establishing a "formal organization" called the Association of University Programs in Hospital Administration (AUPHA, 1948). The group included two representatives from each of the following:

- University of Chicago
- Columbia University
- University of Minnesota
- Northwestern University
- University of Toronto
- Washington University
- Yale University

It also included one guest representing the W.K. Kellogg Foundation.

Earnest though they most likely were, the founders could not possibly have foreseen the seismic changes in healthcare the next 70 years would bring. Nor could they have foreseen that those changes would drive the evolution of their association of 15 into a meeting of more than 350 in Philadelphia for the 70th anniversary gathering of the Association of University Programs in Health Administration (AUPHA).

LAYING THE FOUNDATION

Prior to 1948, a handful of university programs met informally. Some, such as the Marquette program, started and then stopped, while others, such as the program at the University of Chicago, demonstrated some degree of staying power (Loebs, 2001). Like the nascent health administration profession itself, the academic underpinning was finding its footing, its mission. The uncertainty about the proper academic home was prominent during the first half of the 20th century, with several of the founders' programs housed in schools of public health, one in business, and one in medicine. The birth of health administration programs predates the advent of schools of allied health or health sciences, which ultimately became the leading home for such programs, along with schools of public health and business.

Practitioners, of course, dominated the early programs. One might suggest that practitioners looking to create academic programs were seeking an academic patina to an otherwise unrecognized line of work. However, they more likely sought an academic foundation for what they knew was an increasingly intricate profession. Whatever attracted the founders to fashioning an academic footing for their work, the movement grew through the middle part of the 20th century. Naturally, as academics became more involved, challenges arose to the intellectual sufficiency of the early programs. Most consisted of one year of didactic education and one year of field placement, raising the question of whether the content rose to the level of *graduate* education. For the programs established before the mid-1960s, the answer was generally yes. In the mid-1960s, however, the two-year didactic model became increasingly prevalent to make room for more content, and many programs substantially reduced their administrative residency requirements. Thus began something of a pendulum swinging between the domination of teaching and mentoring by practitioners and the molding of young professionals by academics. In other words, as the practitioners invaded the academic citadel for validation of their work, the intellectual community subsumed them over time. The traditional rewards associated with life in the academy began to take precedence. Grant funding, publications, and original—as well as applied—research grew within this new field. The federal government rapidly expanded funding for all kinds of research, which benefitted and provided a catalyst to accelerate the growing number of health administration preparation programs. This expanded funding of research assured a small but growing coterie of faculty that there were sufficient resources to win grant funding and advance the knowledge associated with health services research and health services management as well as their careers.

Massive expansion of healthcare began in 1965 with the enactment of Medicare and Medicaid, which brought the need for a greater number of professional administrators and increased the demand for health administration programs.

As the profession grew—some would say in generational waves—so, too, did AUPHA (Loebs, 2001). The association hired its first full-time leader in 1965, Gary Filerman. His long and distinguished tenure created the bedrock for the association. With Filerman's hiring, AUPHA flourished, as he successfully leveraged the compelling story of a growing profession against federal monies and grant dollars to expand association activities. During this era, AUPHA moved from Chicago to Washington, DC, as it took on an advocacy role in addition to curriculum development and providing other services to members. AUPHA also tackled the thorny issues surrounding diversity in the profession and the complex issues of improving health administration on a global scale. The details of those and other stories appear in later chapters and need not be recounted here.

THE MEETING THAT LAUNCHED AN ASSOCIATION

The initial meeting of AUPHA's founders addressed the core question of whether there was a need for an association. The response was a definitive yes. The minutes (AUPHA, 1948) indicate that the group identified five primary reasons for the association:

- An opportunity to discuss common problems
- Setting standards
- Accreditation
- Promoting health administration education leading to a degree
- Development and promotion of research in health administration

Other meeting topics provide clues to the challenges the founders faced in 1948. Interestingly, many of these remain challenges for AUPHA today and became chapters in this book. They include issues such as standard setting, curriculum development, and the need for globalization.

During the meeting, participants directed a group, led by Ray Brown from the University of Chicago, to draft organizational bylaws that would provide strong direction in areas of standards and students. These bylaws dictated many features, including the following.

- Courses (their name for programs) must lead to a master's degree or equivalent.
- Courses must be university based.
- Programs should involve one year of academic instruction followed by one year of residency.
- One-third of the academic portion must be devoted to hospital administration.

Another challenge addressed was competition for students and residency placement. The founders agreed on a common application deadline from April 1 to April 15, with a requirement that students decide on an offer by May 1. Further, no recommendation regarding residency placement could be made by a program until February 1 for the May/June residency year. As reflected in the minutes, the group discussed other issues of general interest reflected in the following list:

- Program size was discussed but left to the discretion of the programs. The size at the time ranged from six students at Yale to 35 at Northwestern.
- Paid residencies were discouraged. A one-year unpaid residency was equivalent to a two-year paid one.
- Residencies in general hospitals were preferred over those in specialty hospitals.
- Preceptors for a residency were evaluated by educational attitude, aptitude, philosophy, and whether the individual was a fellow/member/nominee in the American College of Hospital Administration.
- No specific undergraduate degree was required because the members valued a broad selection.
- Grades were not sufficient for admission; a student needed prior work and an interview.
- The student was required to be between 25 and 35 years old.
- Women were allowed in the program but were noted to be difficult to place.
- People of color were allowed, but they often had jobs to which they could return.

TWO KEY ASPECTS OF AUPHA HISTORY

Although many of the accomplishments, challenges, and defining trends that AUPHA has encountered across its history are detailed in this book, two notable aspects do not appear as individual chapters. They are nonetheless vital to the development of the association and are thus outlined here.

The Canadian Influence

From its infancy, AUPHA was not so much an "American" organization as a "North American" association. During its early days, the concept of a "borderless" AUPHA was prominent. The fact that the University of Toronto was among the founding members laid the groundwork for the proposition that Canadian programs were so closely akin to U.S. ones that looking at them differently would be a distinction without a difference. Our friends in the north were—and remain—important colleagues and peers.

Likewise, the Accrediting Commission on Education for Health Services Administration (ACHESA) (originally ACEGHA)—the first accrediting organization for health services management programs—also took the position that Canadian programs were akin to American ones. The only distinction made during ACHESA site visits was the certainty of including a Canadian practitioner or faculty member when surveying programs in Canada. According to Sherril Gelmon, longtime AUPHA leader, this is unique: No other accrediting organization crosses borders in this way except for Joint Commission International (JCI).

Of the Canadian programs in health management, the University of Toronto has been at the forefront in providing leadership for AUPHA. That first meeting in 1948 included Ms. Eugenie Stuart, a nurse by training, and Dr. L. O. Bradley. Both were responsible for starting the University of Toronto's program. Engagement of other Canadian programs, such as those at the Universities of Alberta, Montreal, British Columbia, and Ottawa, has varied over time. Ryerson University's undergraduate program has been an AUPHA member for many years. Dalhousie University joined the ranks in 1991.

Canadian programs typically were housed in schools of medicine, though the Ottawa program was part of the school of business, where it competed with the MBA program. Perhaps even more than American programs, the Canadian ones were resource-constrained. The provincial governments, according to AUPHA stalwart Peggy Leatt, would not allow programs to keep tuition money. This practice forced them to live within the limited means provided by their various universities, with no incentive to grow enrollment and no reward for extending the educational product to others. Thus, for some of the Canadian programs, participation in AUPHA and ACHESA (now the Commission on Accreditation of Healthcare Management Education, or CAHME) has waxed and waned due to limited resources combined with the inflated costs associated with those activities when translated to Canadian dollars.

Canada has provided several AUPHA leaders:

◆ G. Harvey Agnew, MD, was chair of the AUPHA Board from 1953 to 1954.
◆ University of Montreal physician Dr. Gerald LaSalle chaired the Board from 1963 to 1964.
◆ Another physician, Dr. Burns Roth, was chair from 1969 to 1970.
◆ Peggy Leatt, who was the first female Board chair, served from 1987 to 1988.
◆ Ross Baker, hailing from the Toronto program, was the last chair from Canada, from 2002 to 2004.

During the 1980s and 1990s, Canadian programs were universally included on various task forces regarding curriculum development and faculty development, and also led several symposia. Ross Baker's membership on the Pew Task Force on Quality Improvement in Health Management Education from 1989 to 1992 led to his becoming Board chair a few years later.

Collaborations: The Influence of Partners

During AUPHA's development, it collaborated with many other organizations, including but not limited to the following:

- American Hospital Association (AHA)
- Medical Group Management Association (MGMA)
- Healthcare Information and Management Systems Society (HIMSS)
- Healthcare Financial Management Association (HFMA)
- AcademyHealth (AH)
- International Hospital Federation (IHF)
- Health Administration Press (HAP) (This partnership is addressed in a subsequent chapter.)

Perhaps, however, the most important and durable partnership AUPHA has had over the years is with the American College of Healthcare Executives (ACHE). The American College of Healthcare Executives is an international professional society of 40,000 healthcare executives who lead hospitals, healthcare systems, and other healthcare organizations. ACHE's mission is to advance its members and healthcare management excellence. This coincides closely with AUPHA's mission; thus, it is natural for the two organizations to work closely in preparing future leaders. The author gratefully acknowledges the contributions of Tom Dolan for assisting with the development of the sidebar on ACHE and AUPHA together.

ACHE and AUPHA Together

ACHE and AUPHA have a rich history of collaboration, face some challenges today, but expect a bright future together. The collaboration potential results from a realization that academics and practitioners make a strong team in preparing leaders. Every program needs core faculty with the requisite academic credentials who can teach relevant content and help students develop necessary competencies. Practitioners in the classroom provide valuable orientation to the healthcare industry, however. It is important to get students out into the field of practice, so they can better understand real-world settings and problems. The most valuable experiences for students are internships and fellowships, as these become pipelines for students' future career opportunities. The practitioners in the classroom and opportunities for internships and fellowships evolved from the historical bonds formed by ACHE and AUPHA.

Joint leadership facilitated the historical productive relationship between ACHE and AUPHA. Richard Stull, Stuart Wesbury, and Tom Dolan, former leaders of ACHE, all chaired the AUPHA Board during their careers. Consequently, there was clear alignment of goals and initiatives between the organizations. The relationship continues today but has become more complicated as the constituencies of the two organizations diverged. ACHE and AUPHA must work to determine what each organization could do with and for the other.

Many challenges confront both organizations today as they strive to prepare leaders for the healthcare industry. There will continue to be rapid change in the healthcare industry, as we have seen in the past. While the subject of many conversations, papers, and other communications, some of the key items that ACHE and AUPHA will face in the future are addressed in this volume:

- ◆ Undergraduate and graduate education must reflect the field. Change is occurring quickly, and the curriculum must respond to the change in how society views healthcare, access to services, governmental versus individual responsibility, science, pharma, genomics, treatment processes, and management information systems, among other topics. We must impress upon students the importance of lifelong learning, which involves their reading set, business publications, and general news, and how it applies to their roles in the profession. Chapter 10 on evidence-based management addresses this challenge directly. Also, Chapter 3 addresses the decision to expand AUPHA by including undergraduate programs, in part, as a response to industry pressure.
- ◆ Competencies enhance the educational outcome. Competencies must become integral to all educational programs. Courses in business, healthcare organization, and government must prepare students to deal with change, and students need to learn to work effectively in teams. Naturally, not all competency attainment occurs in the formal educational component of learning. Students must understand the value of lifelong learning. Competencies can be a challenge to define formally and reliably measure, but just because something is difficult

(continued)

to measure does not mean we should not try. Chapter 4 takes on competencies in the context of evaluation and standard setting.

- ◆ We must support women and minorities in academia and practice. There needs to be a continuum of activities to support women and minorities in and out of academia, and these activities need to carry forward in the broader employment market. Leaders must place more emphasis on making sure organizations are diverse and inclusive, including their boards of directors. There has been an emphasis on initial recruitment, but we must do more to keep women and minorities in the pipeline and advance them to middle management and beyond. The industry has to focus its diversity and inclusion initiatives for 10 years following recruitment of women and minorities to see what happens to them and how their tenure in an organization advances. Talented women and minorities leave the field because they cannot advance beyond middle management. Chapter 5 examines these and related issues.

Going forward, many believe that we will see more change in the industry in the next decade than we did over the last 50 years. Diagnosis-related groups were a significant development in the 1980s. There was a commitment to maintain the beneficial features of Medicare and Medicaid. The challenge now is to continue improving the healthcare system. Fifty years ago, there was an emphasis on providing unlimited amounts of care. This, in the eyes of many, is a philosophy we can no longer afford. Leaders need to develop and implement healthcare that is, in the words from the Institute of Medicine, safe, effective, timely, patient-oriented, efficient, and equitable. There will be more public debate about a single-payer system, how care is to be delivered, and by whom. Population health will increasingly become a focus among many other issues such as chronic disease management, the continued migration of care from inpatient to outpatient settings, and access to appropriate care at the appropriate time.

The key will be for ACHE and AUPHA, along with all of the other organizations involved in training and delivering care, to continue to work together. Efficiency implies that we leverage our resources to achieve our common goals of improving the quality of care, expanding access to it, and finding ways to mitigate its burgeoning cost.

CONCLUSION

The founding days of AUPHA are certainly significant. Likewise, the partnerships and collaborations with other organizations deserve attention, as those relationships have been a critical part of AUPHA's history. For the 70 years of the association's existence, it has seen and influenced a host of issues and cultural turns. The following pages detail those experiences, allowing us to learn from what has gone before and prepare for the future.

ACKNOWLEDGMENT

The author is especially grateful to Tom Dolan for his intellectual contributions to this chapter.

REFERENCES

Association of University Programs in Health Administration. (1948). *Minutes of the first meeting of the Association of University Programs in Hospital Administration*. New York, NY: Author.

Loebs, S. (2001). The continuing evolution of health management education. *Journal of Health Administration Education*, Special Issue, 33–50.

ABOUT THE AUTHOR

Michael R. Meacham, JD, is an Associate Professor of Health Leadership and Management at the Medical University of South Carolina. He was a member of the Health Policy and Administration faculty at The Pennsylvania State University from 2003 to 2010 and served as Director of the MHA Program. Previously, Mr. Meacham had served as Vice President for Integrated Health Services at the Eastern Connecticut Health Network, as Director of Health System Development for Connecticut's Office of Healthcare Access, and as a member of the Kansas House of Representatives from 1977 until 1985.

CHAPTER 2

The Influence of Academic Location on Health Administration Graduate Programs

Stephen F. Loebs, PhD, and Michael R. Meacham, JD

INTRODUCTION

There has been long-standing contention among academic leaders, as well as national experts, on the appropriate university location for a graduate program in health administration. This contention has not been dominant, but it has occupied dialogue space. Nowhere is this more apparent than in the underpinnings of the Association of University Programs in Health Administration (AUPHA).

Representatives of seven university-based graduate programs located in four distinct academic locations were responsible for starting the association (AUPHA, n.d.). The universities and the schools where the programs were located included the following:

- University of Chicago—School of Business
- Northwestern University—School of Commerce
- Columbia University—School of Public Health
- University of Minnesota—School of Public Health
- University of Toronto—School of Hygiene
- Washington University—School of Medicine
- Yale University—Department of Public Health in School of Medicine

The variation in how these entities opted to house their health administration programs invites several questions: How did the different options come about? How does the variation affect AUPHA and the graduate education field? Do the various locations influence graduate education outcomes and health services management differently? This chapter aims to address some of these questions, providing a history of the variations on the different academic locations, and a discussion of factors that appear to have influenced the various choices.

THE ROLE OF THE FOUNDERS IN THE DEBATE

The amazing collaboration of several key individuals from the seven universities established the tone and direction for AUPHA and various graduate programs:

- Michael Davis, University of Chicago
- Arthur Bachmeyer, University of Chicago
- Malcolm T. MacEachern, Northwestern University
- Harvey T. Agnew, University of Toronto
- Frank Bradley, Washington University
- George Buis, Yale University
- Dwight Barnett, Columbia University
- James A. Hamilton, University of Minnesota

These individuals came from different corners of their respective universities and the field of practice as a whole. Many of the founders and visionaries had mixed academic credentials, dividing their time between two roles: university hospital director and initial program director. Not only were they AUPHA's trailblazers, but they also led the way for the specialized field of hospital administration (now known as health administration), establishing precedents that many have followed. The label *academic entrepreneurs* fits nicely, as these action-oriented individuals were the catalysts and academic risk-takers, defining a credible field of academic endeavor and establishing a new national organization to support it.

Equally important, the founders were bridge builders within their respective universities. Because the programs did not fit neatly into any of the traditional academic departments or schools, the founders needed to be creative to secure a location for their graduate programs, employing opportunism along with networking and a heavy dose of practicality. They negotiated arrangements with key stakeholders to establish their graduate programs, even though the field of study was relatively unknown and unproven. The result was that their programs did not follow any defined prescription—they were located in different places depending on the bridges the founders built.

THE PART FOUNDATIONS PLAYED

The founders did not act alone; the following foundations provided financial support and guidance:

- W.K. Kellogg Foundation
- Rockefeller Foundation

- Rosenwald Fund
- Johnson & Johnson Research Foundation

The Kellogg Foundation was especially influential at the time and in subsequent years, influencing discussions about academic location. Foundation support reflected the interests of a specific foundation. This support is a key element in AUPHA history and in the history of most graduate programs from the mid-1940s to the early 1970s.

CONTENDING MODELS FOR UNIVERSITY LOCATION

When AUPHA approved its constitution and bylaws in 1949, there was no reference to the academic location of member programs within the respective universities—the concept of different locations was accepted. This seemingly established a fundamental tenet: There has always been variation in university location throughout the field's evolution.

Although neither AUPHA nor the accrediting agencies adopted a policy on the topic, strong opinions and differences were expressed from some sources in the first 25 years of the field. In this context, the feelings of early leaders were very public. These differences were generally framed as advocacy for a business school or public health location. These views contained different orientations to graduate education. Neither of these options appear to have dominated in the long run, although schools of public health were apparently the most preferred in the early years. Plus, there was never an advocacy for a medical school–based home.

Starting in the early 1980s, many new graduate programs were located in schools of health professions and allied health, which generally focus on a combination of population health and the other approaches.

Educational content, of course, reflects the academic location and orientation of the program. Each approach contains curriculum content that is generally applicable to a point of emphasis. That said, health administration education requires a hybrid approach to include content across a broad spectrum of academic subjects. How to arrange for and provide for this hybrid is at the crossroads of contention and differences on an appropriate academic home.

A summary of the two original approaches—the business approach and public health approach—as well as attempts at finding the right hybrid can be helpful to understanding the form and shape of graduate education in the current era.

The national discussion on appropriate university location began with the consideration for location employed by Michael Davis in his initiative during the period 1933 to 1934; this was when he established the program at the University of Chicago. Many credit the University of Chicago's School of Business as starting the first enduring graduate program. It was the only program of its kind for about 10 years. After weighing the advantages and theoretical rationale for a location in the medical school, Davis (1959) selected the business school. He stated,

> We placed the hospital administration course under the business school for purely practical reasons . . . lack of interest on the part of the medical faculty, despite opinions of key university leaders that the essential objective of hospital administration was medical not business. . . . [T]o place the hospital administration course under the medical school would be theoretically correct but practically stupid.

The University of Chicago did not have a school of public health at the time, so Davis's options were limited. The criteria Davis used emphasized practicality and recognition of political influence within the university. Many who followed him employed similar criteria.

The period 1945 to 1958, starting 11 years after the University of Chicago opened its program's doors, is particularly important in the annals of graduate health administration education. As referenced previously, program leaders organized AUPHA in 1949. The number of graduate programs expanded rapidly after this point. Also during this period, two nationally based commissions on hospital administration education produced reports that are generally considered special markers for the field. The *Prall Report* (Prall, 1948) and the *Olsen Report* (Olsen, 1954), named after the directors of the study groups that produced them, included discussions and recommendations on university location.

The *Prall Report* gave an endorsement, though guarded, of the importance of schools of public health as preferred locations. Part of this position was reflective of the preference, at the time, of the report's sponsor, the W.K. Kellogg Foundation. There was interest in the potential of fusing instruction in hospital administration with training in health department administration. The *Prall Report*'s authors were not totally convinced this fusion would work but gave the nod of approval to schools of public health. In addition, the report asserted,

> From the beginning the Kellogg Foundation had given priority to requests for program support coming from universities with public health schools. Of the new programs established during the life of the Report, all but one was set up within a school of public health or with joint sponsorship. (Prall, 1958)

The Kellogg Foundation's support for establishing and sustaining graduate education in health administration started in1946. Initial support went to six graduate programs, five of which were located in schools of public health. Kellogg staff explained that the decisions for support in the initial investment were based on the opportunity to have the biggest impact in a short time (Pattullo, 1959). The need for expediency stemmed from a commitment to expand the pool of trained hospital administrators as a result of demand and to take advantage of a large exodus of military personnel at the end of World War II. As such, the programs receiving financial support from Kellogg were already accepting new students or were able to start with a short ramp-up. The precise explanations for the Kellogg support decisions cannot be retrieved, but it is likely that schools of public health were eager to accept graduate programs in health administration with the accompanying financial inducements. The Kellogg Foundation expanded its financial support criteria after the first wave of support.

The *Olsen Report*, published in 1954, was the product of an independent commission created by AUPHA and financed by the Kellogg Foundation. This report was more specific than the *Prall Report* on the topic of academic location. It stated:

> It is clear that there is no one perfect locus for a program in hospital administration and that the program in hospital administration can operate acceptably in any of the schools, such as graduate school, public administration, medicine, public health, business, if the proper arrangements are made with the parent school and if the right people are the administrative officers . . . schools of business administration most nearly approximate the educational content considered desirable for the ideal program with its emphasis on management and administration. (Olsen, 1954, pp. 89, 159)

The contrast of the two reports' conclusions is stark, from quite neutral to very specific. The latter conclusion was the most important for *Olsen*. Stakeholders were not uniform in their support at the time. In fact, the endorsement of the business school as a location for health administration was controversial. AUPHA Board members had heated discussions about emphasis on management and administration. The controversy almost broke up the association, according to one source (Stephan, 1959). The division of opinion centered on the relative emphasis that was to be given to administrative theory and practice as opposed to the environment in which administration takes place. There were two factions, depending on whether the program director's training was in medicine or administration. These factions apparently negotiated an agreement. Although the Board did not accept the *Olsen Report*, the American Council on Education published it. Both sides of stakeholders, passionate in their advocacy, established the boundaries of the debate, making them more clearly defined than at any previous time. Except for the tense time in the AUPHA Board, the conflict did not affect any movements within the field.

One moment during a presentation by Michael Davis at a national symposium in 1958 might have framed the national debate. He referred to the bases of a significant conundrum:

whether the major emphasis in the training of the hospital manager should be on internal administration, as in the usual business enterprise, or on responsibility to the community for management of a comprehensive health program, including hospital services as one of its major facets. (Davis, 1959)

He framed the two emphases as between a business model and a community health model. The community health model was his explicit choice at the time, 25 years after he started the University of Chicago program in a business school for temporal pragmatic reasons.

Finding a proper location for his community health model was apparently elusive for Davis. He was searching for the most appropriate location but not happy with the public health school option. He observed that

the choice of a school of public health for location has even more theoretical appropriateness than medical school auspices. . . . Unhappily the schools of public health rarely measured up to their opportunities . . . They have shown little flexibility in adapting educational programs to the needs of particular fields. (Davis, 1959)

This observation is now about 60 years old, and it should be weighed against current policies of schools of public health. These schools have proven to be willing hosts for the largest number of graduate programs. Davis might change his mind with this evidence.

There have been several other markers, studies, and publications since the previously cited reports and commentary. This historical review should take cognizance of them. In 1972, the Kellogg Foundation continued its sponsorship and commitment for improvement in health administration education by financing a commission to produce an in-depth examination of health administration education. The commission published its findings in 1974 in the *Dixon–Austin Report*, named after the chair of the commission and the major author. This report, like the others, has broad distribution. Its recommendations focused on curriculum content, educational initiatives for practitioners, and student recruitment. These recommendations did not include any reference to appropriate graduate program location.

After release of the *Dixon–Austin Report*, there was reduced public dialogue among stakeholders on the location topic. An exception was a *Report on Education for Health Administration: Issues and Alternatives*, published in November 1980. This report summarized a study under the auspices of the Health Resources Administration of the Department of Health and Human Services (Levey, 1980). It referred to the differences between a business model and a medical model for a graduate program curriculum. It also acknowledged that the balance between models was complicated. The recommendation was that

> emphasis be placed on a balanced curriculum but that it is exceedingly difficult to provide curriculum balance outside the business school model. An important feature should be bridge building with business schools because of the small critical mass of most programs . . . . [L]inkages with other units in relation to future viability should be examined. (Levey, 1980)

It is difficult to trace the impact of these recommendations. On the other hand, they appear to mirror previous observations, they resonate with contemporary challenges, and they reflect a continued searching for the right place.

Alfred P. Sloan Foundation Legacy: The First Two-Year Academic Masters Model at Cornell University

Brooke Hollis

Alfred P. Sloan—former head of General Motors and an avid philanthropist—has been heralded as one of the greatest business leaders of the 20th century. He is known for revolutionizing the auto industry, but his foresight stretched beyond cars. It was his vision of professionally managed hospitals that led to the creation of Cornell's Sloan Program.

In fact, Sloan was thinking about his own demise when he first suggested the idea of creating a school for hospital administrators at Cornell. It was the early 1950s, and then-Cornell President Deane Malott had visited Sloan to inquire about donations to Cornell's College of Engineering.

Sloan told Malott he had not considered donating to Cornell Engineering. In his memoirs in the Cornell archives, Malott wrote, "Then turning to me, he said, 'But I'll tell you something. I expect to die in a hospital someday, and they are very poorly administered.'"

"You at Cornell have a Hotel School, and a hospital is really a specialized kind of hotel," Sloan told Malott. "I've been thinking that hospital administrators should be better trained" (Hall, 2009, p. 1).

(continued)

Sloan agreed to endow a program to train hospital administrators, and the nation's first two-year academic graduate program in hospital administration was born in 1955. That idea later became the dominant model for training health executives until the present day (Haddock, McLean, & Chapman, 2001).

Sloan reportedly became interested in health in part due to his brother Raymond, who for 20 years was president and director of the Modern Hospital in Chicago and editor of its publication, which later became the widely read *Modern Healthcare* ("Raymond P. Sloan," 1983). Raymond Sloan was also a pioneer in examining the role of facilities' design and color in hospitals, authoring a book on the subject. Other notable philanthropic gifts by Alfred Sloan in healthcare and education were for the Memorial Sloan Kettering Cancer Center in New York and the Sloan School of Management at Massachusetts Institute of Technology.

Over the years, Sloan's prescient idea that hospitality and healthcare had a link has gained much more recognition, especially with the advent of the Hospital Consumer Assessment of Healthcare Providers and Systems surveys, which look at patient experience and link them to reimbursement, and the adoption of evidence-based design ideas to improve health facilities (Hines, Luna, Marquardt, & Stelmokas, 2008; Taylor, 2012). Cornell has long had close relationships with the Hotel School and Sloan Program. More recently, it has formalized these with a two-school Institute for Healthy Futures, which explores innovations across health, hospitality, and design—mirroring many of the ideas of the two Sloan brothers who inspired the creation of the graduate program at Cornell that bears the Sloan name (Mulconry, 2016; Weed, 2016).

DISTRIBUTION BY ACADEMIC LOCATION

Baseline information on the evolution of academic locations provides a reference for understanding the current state of location variation. After the University of Chicago created its program, 11 more universities established programs from 1943 to 1950. Here is a breakdown of the different programs and the schools in which they were housed (Loebs, 2001):

Type of school	Number	Percent of total
Public Health	7	63
Graduate	2	18
Business	1	9
Medicine	1	9

Several factors could explain the relative dominance by public health schools, including the influence of foundations and the degree of compatibility that these schools offered.

Today there are 10 different academic homes for full-time AUPHA-member health administration graduate programs in the United States and Canada (G. Glandon, personal communication, November 4, 2017). Here is the current breakdown:

Type of school	Number	Percent of total
Public Health	25	33
Health Professions or Allied Health	25	33
Business	20	20
Public Policy and Public Administration	3	4
Other (includes five locations)	5	5
Medicine	2	3

In looking at the tables, several questions emerge:

1. What prompted the expansion of program homes from four to ten?
2. What are the differences in the input characteristics among the programs, such as the characteristics of matriculating students?
3. What are the early and long-term career paths of graduating students?
4. What are the differences among programs with similar university locations?

There are no global answers or explanations for the abovementioned questions. Instead, the answers reside in each program's individual history and information.

Note that the growth in numbers and locations occurred without any external constraints, and the actual number of programs is likely higher, as many graduate programs are not AUPHA affiliated. In addition, the growth of external degree programs, executive programs, and online options add considerably to the graduate program terrain. There are additional organizational configurations and concentrations in health administration, generally located in schools of business and schools of public health. They award graduate degrees associated with their schools, sometimes with an attached specialty identification, such as an MBA in Health Administration.

Clearly, universities have responded in different ways to the expanding interest in and demands for better-prepared hospital administrators since World War II. There were no specific guidelines or requirements for location at the time of the early founders. Further, there have never been regulations or laws that dictate the source of an administrator's degree. There is no empirical evidence that one location is dominant or better. Anyone trying to figure out the differences among graduate programs and trying to choose among them—especially with regard to academic location—is confronted with a wall of confusion and an absence of any useful, objective guidelines.

CHALLENGES TO INTEGRATION WITHIN UNIVERSITIES

As mentioned earlier in this chapter, idiosyncratic factors at each university provide the primary explanations for academic location decisions. Although these explanations are unique, they are unfortunately somewhat rare, as only a few programs have produced histories that include the rationale underlying their academic home. Nevertheless, there are some common denominators regarding the challenges faced by program founders both in the early days and at present. These themes include the following:

- *The programs' small size.* The attribute of small size narrowed the options for location in the early years. In some cases, the number of students and faculty in the program did not support an autonomous unit. The programs also had limited funds, few qualified faculty, no alumni support, and limited leverage as virtual start-ups. In these situations, an attractive option was to fold a graduate program into an existing unit. That said, many programs in the first generation and beyond had the attraction of external funds to open the doors. This availability could have neutralized initial concerns about financing a start-up, regardless of size.
- *An uneasy fit for the newness of an untried and unknown program.* Graduate education in health administration is not a neat fit, if at all, in a traditional academic area or in existing professional schools. There are multiple subject needs covering a broad continuum of foci from business to medical care to public health to the social sciences. There was no history of a usual and customary location for an atypical set of academic interests.
- *Disputes about the importance of values manifested by different perspectives.* A basic question that emerged was, what are the graduate programs educating students to do? Should a school have more of a social science orientation or a business orientation or a community health orientation? The answer could range from managing hospitals to managing public health departments. Participants have muted these disputes in recent years, perhaps in implicit recognition that there is no one "right" combination. Universities and programs will tailor their respective orientations to address perceived local and regional needs.

- *Focus on an industry, not a defined academic discipline.* There was minimal reference or experience in the universities with a program that focused on an industry and a social problem. Unlike the venerable professions of law and medicine, health administration was more of an amalgamation of disciplines rather than a discrete subject of study.

Beyond the challenges described in the preceding list, program founders coped with a set of specific administrative hurdles in search of a location. These hurdles were daunting; they had to find an academic home that would provide access to basic requirements, such as space, classrooms, and library facilities. They had to identify an academic host with whom they shared common interests. They had to find a location that could provide access to relevant graduate-level courses and a graduate degree within a specified time. A valuable resource was a colleague who could navigate the existing university protocols. The degree of success in overcoming these hurdles most probably led to the decision on location for the graduate program. No one could share a map for finding a common fit because there was none.

NO MEASURE OF OUTCOMES

No published evidence compares the outcomes of graduate programs located in different academic settings, nor is there evidence on the outcomes tied to completing different core course requirements. In other words, no one knows with any certainty if one location or set of required courses makes for more complete student preparation than others. This leads to the supposition that accreditors' recent emphasis on mission-based competencies may be an approach borne of this uncertainty.

The Commission on Accreditation of Healthcare Management Education (CAHME) provides evidence of a program's ability to meet a quality baseline by successfully applying content and competency criteria to a program's mission-defined elements. Historically, availability of information about program-specific accreditation elements has been limited, defying meaningful comparison between programs. Current changes in accreditation-related reporting may yield salient change in this circumstance.

The most recent initiative to bring together national leaders in health administration practice and education to discuss the future occurred in 2001 at the National Summit on the Future of Education and Practice in Health Management and Policy (Authors, 2001). One of the long-term outcomes of this conference has been the restructuring of the accreditation process. One outcome pushed CAHME to become more than just an accreditation council, as its mission focused on enhancing the quality of graduate healthcare management education. For example, as required in its accrediting standards, CAHME mandates that programs supply key measures indicative of program strength, including admission standards, yield of matriculated students to applicants, student retention rates, graduate placement rates, and core curriculum requirements, among other measures. CAHME's website was reconfigured and will make these data available to the public as required by the Council for Higher Education Accreditation (CHEA) in the first quarter of 2018 (A. Stanowski, personal communication, December 27, 2017).

The gap in meaningful comparison information means there is no way to form an evidence-based judgment on the outcomes of comparing one graduate program with others. It is impossible to obtain any centrally located or published information about the programs presented in a common template. Although data such as percentage of employment and types of placement do exist, there is no empirical method for determining that one academic location is relatively "better." Stakeholders can, however, make reasonably informed judgments about the suitability of a program for their particular needs.

The absence of meaningful, comparative information has sometimes created a vacuum replaced with hyperbole, unsubstantiated boasting, speculation, and institutionally based claims of excellence. Applicants to the graduate programs and potential employers need to discern this issue for themselves.

Although an examination of the importance and relevancy of academic location may appear warranted, broad-based evaluation would be complex and potentially volatile—not to mention the academic rewards may be limited. An objective, evidence-based evaluation of outcome differences based on academic location does not appear to be on the horizon.

THE IMPACT ON AUPHA

For AUPHA, the diversity of locations has presented some challenges. Searching for a common denominator to maintain programmatic and organizational commitment was and continues to be a nuanced endeavor. Oftentimes, program representatives from different university locations have had different obligations and preferences for external validation, such as overlapping accreditation. Overall, the diversity in program locations can produce dissonance and is a reality with which AUPHA must continue to wrestle.

On the other hand, there have been some advantages to the location disparities. Various academic affiliations, each with different histories and perspectives, create the unique, eclectic consortium of AUPHA members. In fact, this is one of AUPHA's distinguishing characteristics, not to mention what sets the field of graduate health administration education apart from other academic disciplines. The mix of members with different preferences and biases, plus the individual leaders with vastly different resumes, have provided a plethora of perspectives and preferences at the policy table. In addition, the different course and experiential requirements have presented a mix of choices for applicants, faculty employment, and potential employers.

CONCLUSION

Since the formative years of graduate health administration education, stakeholders have posited the relative merits of several academic locations. From the initial days of AUPHA and the first generation of graduate programs, the predominant variables to affect location have been the response to university political factors, the welcome mat offered by leaders of existing university units, encouragement and direct influence by foundations, and direct and probably aggressive approaches to segments of the universities by program founders. Any one of these or a combination, together with gradual solutions to the challenges cited above, provide the explanations for variation.

The reports of three national commissions and related reports, concentrated in a period from the late 1940s to mid-1980s, reflect interest in this subject. These reports and summits have helped to define the pros and cons of competing approaches for curriculum and location. They have not led to a consensus at the national level. On the other hand, graduate programs have emerged with many of the attributes suggested by the national attention. This focus has clearly had influence, but the lack of consensus and lack of documented evidence on the effectiveness of the competing approaches mutes the debate.

There is continued interest in the significance of the local variations. The stimuli for this interest are manifold. First, keen competition from new forms of access to graduate education, such as external degree programs and long-distance learning, emanates from diverse academic settings. Second, other graduate programs that interpret an attractive market for their offerings perpetuate local variations. Third, changing sets of skills defined by an expanding group of potential employers for competence in entry-level and senior management positions encourage continual curricula redevelopment. Finally, the cost of graduate education motivates leaders to compress content and competency development as much as possible. These stimuli influence all graduate programs, regardless of university location.

The current variation in graduate program location, with 10 different locations within university structures, does make a difference in outcomes for students, alumni, faculty, and potential employers as to appropriate preparation for a given market.

No one knows with objective certainty, however, which approach is qualitatively "better" than another. The best approach may be different for each key stakeholder group. It may be different as a function of mission. It may be different within the organizational structure of the university. In the absence of any centrally located and evidence-based comparison of graduate program locations, each location's outcomes must be determined on its own merits, with reference to its mission and supporting evidence of its individual outcomes. The outcomes are multifaceted, with multiple stakeholders.

The value of one location versus another cannot and should not be assessed without reference to the contributions to improvement of population health, financing and delivery of comprehensive health services, and quality of outcomes. While the contributions may not be direct and personal, they can be made by many levers at the disposal of faculty, students, and alumni. The evidence of these contributions reveals the true fabric of the programs.

ACKNOWLEDGMENTS

The authors gratefully acknowledge the valuable recommendations for this chapter from Sharon Schweikhart, Gary Filerman, and Anthony Kovner.

REFERENCES

Association of University Programs in Health Administration (AUPHA). (n.d.). History of AUPHA. Retrieved from: http://www.aupha.org/about/history

Authors, M. (2001). *The future of education and practice in health management and policy: Proceedings from the National Summit*. Orlando, FL: AUPHA.

Davis, M. (1959). Development of the first graduate program in hospital administration. In R. Brown (Ed.), *Graduate education for hospital administration* (pp. 6–21). Chicago, IL: University of Chicago.

Haddock, C. C., McLean, R. A., & Chapman, R. C. (2001). *Careers in healthcare management*. Chicago, IL: Health Administration Press. Retrieved from www.ache.org/healthmanagementcareers/haddock_ch01.pdf

Hall, S. (2009, April 20). Sloan program to graduate its 50th class this May. *Cornell Chronicle*. Retrieved from http://news.cornell.edu/stories/2009/04/sloan-program-graduate-its-50th-class-may

Hines, S., Luna, K., Lofthus, J., Marquardt, M., & Stelmokas, D. (2008). *Becoming a high reliability organization: Operational advice for hospital leaders* (AHRQ Publication No. 08-0022, prepared by the Lewin Group under Contract No. 290-04-0011). Retrieved from https://archive.ahrq.gov/professionals/quality-patient-safety/quality-resources/tools/hroadvice/hroadvice.pdf

Levey, S. (1980). *Education for health administration: Issues and alternatives.* Washington, DC: Department of Health and Human Services.

Loebs, S. (2001). The continuing evolution of health management education. *Journal of Health Administration Education* (Special Issue), 33–50.

Mulconry, S. (2016, Spring). A design for better, more hospitable care. *Hotelie.* Retrieved from https://blogs.cornell.edu/healthyfutures/files/2016/07/CIHF-Hotelie-article-y8eraj.pdf

Olsen, H. (1954). *University education for administration of hospitals: A report of the Commission on University Education in Hospital Administration.* Washington, DC: American Council on Education.

Pattullo, A. (1959). Foundations and their role in the development of graduate education in hospital administration. In R. Brown (Ed.), *Graduate education for hospital administration* (pp. 58–67). Chicago, IL: University of Chicago.

Prall, C. (1948). *The college curriculum in hospital administration: A final report by the Joint Commission on Education.* Chicago, IL: Physicians' Record Company.

Prall, C. (1958). A review of the report of the Joint Commission on Education for Hospital Administration. In R. Brown (Ed.), *Graduate education for hospital administration* (pp. 29–42). Chicago, IL: University of Chicago.

Raymond P. Sloan dies at 90; Hospital management expert. (1983, March 23). *The New York Times.* Retrieved from www.nytimes.com/1983/03/23/obituaries/raymond-p-sloan-dies-at-90-hospital-management-expert.html

Stephan, J. (1959). The development of the Association of University Programs in Hospital Administration. In R. Brown (Ed.), *Graduate education for hospital administration* (pp. 68–73). Chicago, IL: University of Chicago.

Taylor, E. (2012, September 6). Evidence-based design and the Pebble Project: 12 years later. *Healthcare Design.* Retrieved from http://www.healthcaredesignmagazine.com/trends/architecture/evidence-based-design-and-pebble-project-12-years/

Weed, J. (2016, August 1). With room service and more, hospitals borrow from hotels. *The New York Times.* Retrieved from https://www.nytimes.com/2016/08/02/business/making-hospitals-more-like-hotels.html

ABOUT THE AUTHORS

Stephen F. Loebs, PhD, is Professor Emeritus of Health Services Management and Policy, College of Public Health, The Ohio State University, and Research Associate, Bowdoin College. He was a member of the faculty of the Graduate Program in Health Services and Management at The Ohio State University from 1972 to 2010 and served as Chair of the Graduate Program from 1980 to 2002. He is a Filerman Prize recipient. The Ohio State University established an Endowed Professorship in his name.

Michael R. Meacham, JD, is an Associate Professor of Health Leadership and Management at the Medical University of South Carolina. He was a member of the Health Policy and Administration faculty at The Pennsylvania State University from 2003 to 2010 and served as Director of the MHA Program. Previously, Mr. Meacham had served as Vice President for Integrated Health Services at the Eastern Connecticut Health Network, as Director of Health System Development for Connecticut's Office of Healthcare Access, and as a member of the Kansas House of Representatives from 1977 until 1985.

CHAPTER 3

The Historic Shift in AUPHA's Mission and Membership: Undergraduate Programs Join the Association

Lee F. Seidel, PhD

INTRODUCTION

The inclusion of undergraduate programs in the Association of University Programs in Health Administration (AUPHA) was a significant event in the association's history, and in the history of undergraduate health administration programs. This story, while full of twists and turns, resulted in undergraduate programs earning full AUPHA membership.

In retrospect, initially there was outright opposition to incorporating undergraduate programs. However, they were eventually included, albeit with tepid acceptance at first and a relationship that was a work in progress. Passion characterized both the supporters and opponents of this effort. Prior to becoming a part of the association, undergraduate programs challenged the status quo of AUPHA.

This chapter tells the story of how undergraduate programs became part of AUPHA. It also memorializes those individuals who led and influenced the process of changing the association's mind-set and bringing the programs into the fold. Using interviews, AUPHA Board minutes, and other published works, the chapter includes the author's conclusions concerning specific factors that contributed to the original union between undergraduate health administration education and AUPHA. This chapter discusses several issues, acknowledging that some are still relevant today.

THE ORIGINS OF THE UNDERGRADUATE PROGRAM

Although undergraduate programs in health administration existed prior to 1970, they were rare. Some evidence suggests that the first recorded undergraduate program at Marquette University began in 1928, but it was short-lived (Loebs, 2001).

Following that effort, there is clear evidence that Georgia State University began an undergraduate program in the early 1950s. R. C. Williams started the Georgia State University certificate program in the mid-1950s. It then became a bachelor's in business (BBA) program with a health administration major in 1957 and existed until 1980 (A. Sumner, personal communication, February 12, 2014). There may be other pioneers that are now lost in history. Some conclude that the "undergraduate era in health administration" began between 1965 and 1970 (Cohen, 1977; Gordon, 1975). For the sake of this chapter, we start our saga around 1965 and acknowledge that at this time very few operational undergraduate programs existed in higher education.

During this period, undergraduate programs existed to meet local demands and had no national forum or national recognition. At best, they had limited knowledge of similar programs at other academic institutions. Moreover, these academic programs emanated from the specific mission and goals of the institution providing the program, and there were no norms to guide the "undergraduate" program in general. Each early pioneer had a unique story. Note that in this time frame *undergraduate* meant an academic degree program that awarded either the associate's or the bachelor's degree.

THE 89TH CONGRESS: 1965–1967

The modern era of undergraduate health administration began with the 89th Congress (1965–1967) and the enactment of significant federal health-related legislation. This Congress redefined the healthcare sector and its need for educated administrators. For example, in July 1965, Public Law No. 89-97 created Medicare and Medicaid. In November 1966, Congress enacted Public Law No. 89-749 to create the Comprehensive Health Planning and Services Act (subsequently replaced in 1974 by the Health Planning and Resources Development Act). The 89th Congress also developed the Regional Medical Program through Public Law No. 89-239.

Medicare and Medicaid substantially expanded access to care, which redefined the financing of services provided by hospitals, physician practices, and nursing homes. This also brought about the need for administrators to manage systems external to a hospital, such as community planning agencies, nursing homes, and mental health clinics. Thus, the field of healthcare administration slowly began to consider systems of care as well as managing hospitals.

THE BEGINNING OF ACCREDITATION

With the beginning of accreditation in 1968 by the Accrediting Commission on Graduate Education for Hospital Administration (ACGEHA) and its subsequent recognition by the U.S. Office of Education, thereby making federal money available to health administration programs, the question of undergraduate membership in AUPHA became more contentious. Formal accreditation for graduate programs likely was one of the original barriers faced by undergraduate programs. In this era, only the "entry-level degrees for professional practices" were eligible for federally sanctioned accreditation. AUPHA's inability to define how undergraduate programs differed from graduate programs was the source of some of the original opposition to including undergraduate programs. In other words, some in AUPHA did not see a unique role and function for undergraduate programs. The question of the intended competencies associated with the undergraduate degree—in contrast to the graduate degree—was not answered to AUPHA's satisfaction, and many believed that recognition of the undergraduate degree for entry into the professional practice would jeopardize graduate programs' accreditation status. As documented in the AUPHA Board minutes, "The Executive Committee of AUPHA takes the position that within the very near future, all hospitals, other health facilities, and health programs should be administered by individuals with appropriate administrative education at the graduate level" (AUPHA Records, 1968b).

At this time, all full members of AUPHA programs constituted the legislative authority of the association. Each full-member program had one vote. Its Executive Committee (aka Board of Directors) implemented the will of its legislature.

This extract indicates AUPHA's position on a number of relevant issues. From 1968 forward, AUPHA acted primarily to protect the sanctity of accreditation and accredited graduate degree programs as the entry-level degree for professional practice. It was concerned that including undergraduate programs would jeopardize ACGEHA's (later reconstituted as ACEHSA) legitimacy to accredit, thereby ending the hegemony of graduate programs in health and hospital administration. Federal manpower funding also required specialized accreditation. As such, accredited graduate programs in hospital administration also had a significant financial interest in this issue.

The Kellogg Foundation's Impact on the Undergraduate Program Question

As mentioned in previous chapters, the W.K. Kellogg Foundation, along with a number of critical pioneers, provided the vision and support for the development of AUPHA. For decades, the Kellogg Foundation was AUPHA's primary supporter. In their strategic collaboration, the foundation and AUPHA (along

(continued)

with its member academic programs) were originally committed to building a (new) profession—hospital administration. In their collaborative vision, master's degree graduates from AUPHA member programs would manage hospitals. Their professional metaphor was medical education (Filerman, 1983; G. Filerman, personal communication, February 13, 2014). Formal graduate studies in hospital administration were to be followed by internships and residencies. This vision also prioritized collaboration with the American College of Hospital Administrators (ACHA), American Hospital Association (AHA), and the Blue Cross/Blue Shield Association (Filerman, 1983).

The difference between this vision and reality deserves comment. Even with the advent of specialized accreditation in the form of ACEHSA, there is no evidence that the professional societies ever embraced—or officially endorsed—an accredited degree in hospital or health administration as a *required* credential for affiliation and professional practice. Becoming a profession like law or medicine was already a false hope.

The AUPHA/Kellogg vision also prioritized the development of the body of knowledge that would fully develop the profession and contribute to the quality of professional preparation. In 1963, Kellogg's Program Officer Andrew Pattullo indicated "it was time" for programs to enhance cooperation to improve their (individual and collective) quality (G. Filerman, personal communication, February 13, 2014). From this emerged Kellogg's funding for AUPHA curricula task forces, made up of faculty and practitioners, to define curricula standards and resources for graduate-level programs (G. Filerman, personal communication, February 13, 2014). The field also thirsted for well-qualified faculty with doctoral degrees, and the associated research directly focused on hospital management questions and issues. The field also needed textbooks, research articles, and cases based on formal research.

According to Gary Filerman, PhD, AUPHA's first president and CEO, undergraduate academic programs in health administration just did not fit within this vision and AUPHA's developing paradigm; they did not contribute to the field's status or "the developing profession." He also indicated that "undergraduate programs didn't seem to bring much to the table" (G. Filerman, personal communication, February 13, 2014). He did note that Kellogg provided an undergraduate program development grant to Michigan State University's School of Hotel Administration in the late 1950s or early 1960s, probably as part of the foundation's commitment to the state of Michigan. In expressing AUPHA's view of undergraduate programs at this time, Dr. Filerman stated, "They did not bring federal funds to help AUPHA-affiliated programs develop. Also, the

THE IMPETUS FOR CHANGE

Undergraduate programs in health administration became eligible to join AUPHA as full members in 1975. Based on Board minutes, it is clear that this culminated a seven-year period of serious debate around the "undergraduate question."

One of the things driving the association to debate the issue was the 89th Congress passing Public Law No. 89-751, the Allied Health Professions Personnel Training Act of 1966. This legislation created the authority to award program development grants in allied health. As a result, the Educational Development Branch, Division of Associated Health Professions, Public Health Service, issued program development grants to two baccalaureate programs in health administration:

- In 1968, a grant was awarded to Ithaca College
- In 1970, The Pennsylvania State University won a grant to develop a baccalaureate-level program.

These grants and the undergraduate programs they sponsored became the impetus for eventual change in AUPHA.

The Ithaca College Model

In 1967, Ithaca College began studying possible ways it could meet emerging national healthcare needs. The university's formal study recommended an undergraduate program named Administration of Health Services, leading to a bachelor of science degree. The program used existing resources in health and business and linked the program to a liberal arts base. It then added courses and an internship. As stated by the program's founder and director,

An administrator of health services would initially serve as an assistant administrator and, after obtaining additional professional and/or education experience, as an executive of a voluntary health agency, and/or an administrator of hospitals, nursing homes, or other patient care health activities. (Schneeweiss, 1973, p. 4)

The original proposal indicated the program planned to graduate 25 to 30 individuals per year. It also included an extensive analysis of the regional need for this type of program. Aside from receiving the five-year $268,000 grant from the Public Health Service, Ithaca College indicated it also received more than $100,000 from private foundations and corporations and $150,000 in training stipends for its internship program from 1968 to 1973. Professor Stephen M. Schneeweiss served as this program's founding director. He was succeeded a number of years later by Professor Harold Cohen.

In his essay, "Baccalaureate Education in Health Care Administration," published in 1977 (three years after inclusion in AUPHA), Cohen (1977) provided an early review of baccalaureate health administration education. From his perspective, the tensions that existed prior to undergraduate affiliation remained in 1978 (Cohen, 1977). Aside from chairing the Ithaca College program, Cohen was the first undergraduate faculty member elected to the AUPHA Board of Directors and first chair of an AUPHA Task Force on Undergraduate Education. His historic essay appeared in Volume III of the *Dixon–Austin Report* and included commentary by other commission members, including Professor David Starkweather (California, Berkeley).

The Pennsylvania State University Model

The Pennsylvania State University (in University Park, PA) founded its College of Human Development in 1966. Two years later, in keeping with the plan for the new college, it hired Dr. Marshall W. Raffel from professional practice to direct the college's division of biological health and establish a new baccalaureate program in health planning and administration. Raffel stated, "Health agencies and universities across the land were laboring under the handicap of having too few personnel trained in this field" (Hill & Raffel, 1977, p. 4). He also indicated that comprehensive health planning agencies and regional medical programs were targeted employers for graduates (Hill & Raffel, 1977).

This program had its first graduates in 1971 and saw 60 graduates by 1975, with nine full-time faculty members (Hill & Raffel, 1977). The $460,000 federal grant from the Public Health Services began July 1, 1970. This was an approved and functioning baccalaureate-level program before Penn State received the grant.

In a 2011 interview about the grant, Professor Raffel stated:

Some graduate programs sent a joint letter to the Bureau of Health Manpower recommending that the bureau not fund baccalaureate programs. I was in the process of preparing a grant proposal from Penn State, and in discussing the

PSU proposal with the Bureau of Health Manpower when I was instructed to emphasize health planning since Ithaca was funded for administration. I can't help but feel that the approval of my grant was also an in-your-face response to that letter sent by graduate programs. I should mention that John Griffith at Michigan did not sign that letter and strongly felt that the letter sent from graduate programs was unethical. (M. Raffel, personal communication, July 12, 2011)

THE PATH TO AUPHA MEMBERSHIP: 1968–1975

This section offers a micro history of the journey toward AUPHA membership for undergraduate programs. Quotes from minutes and references to them follow the dates of the official AUPHA Board meetings.

1968–1969: AUPHA Recognizes the Issues

As stated, the primary impetus for AUPHA's consideration of the undergraduate question began with the 1968 federal grant to Ithaca College. Almost immediately, discussion of this grant appears in the minutes of the AUPHA Executive Committee (AUPHA Records, 1968a). The committee's discussion was that such training was not appropriate. The Executive Committee asked staff to gather input from all member programs regarding the undergraduate question. An addendum to these minutes (AUPHA Records, 1968b) restated AUPHA's position that "all hospitals and other health sector organizations should be administered by individuals with appropriate administrative training at the graduate level."

The March 1969 AUPHA Executive Committee discussed potential grants involving long-term care and mental health administration, even though AUPHA still used "Hospital Administration" in its official name. The minutes reflect AUPHA's receptivity to consider new initiatives that complemented its mission, goals, and history.

The Executive Committee again discussed the undergraduate question. The committee recognized that admitting undergraduate programs to full membership could cause a problem for the association, but nonetheless saw the issue as worthy of discussion. To include these "new" types of programs would require AUPHA to embrace a number of other forms of education offerings. At this meeting, the Executive Committee decided to open a dialogue with undergraduate programs. It invited representatives from some of these programs to the April 1969 Annual Meeting for a formal discussion.

The attendance list for the April 1969 Annual Meeting shows five undergraduate faculty:

- Professor Theodore Heimarck, representing Concordia College in Minnesota
- Professor W. D. Pederson, representing Concordia College
- Professor George Wren, representing Georgia State University
- Professor Stephen M. Schneeweiss, representing Ithaca College
- Professor Marshall W. Raffel, representing The Pennsylvania State University

In reflecting on this meeting, Raffel reports that Ithaca College's program director specifically asked AUPHA to open its membership to undergraduate programs. Raffel stated:

The board was obviously negative, continuing to argue against BS programs. At that point I joined the discussion and stated that we had the money, some faculty already on board, and that we were going ahead whether AUPHA liked it or not, and that I wasn't even sure PSU would join if membership was available. (M. Raffel, personal communication, July 12, 2011)

1970: Issues and an Action Plan

In March 1970, the Executive Committee agreed that undergraduate programs were here to stay and decided, formally, to "consider" bachelor-level programs for membership (AUPHA Records, 1970a). The logic was simple. Undergraduate programs were not going away, and working with them inside the AUPHA framework could benefit the field and the association more than undergraduate programs starting their own association.

The Executive Committee planned a fall 1970 meeting with academic program directors to review a proposed amendment to the AUPHA Constitution and Bylaws. At this point, the association anticipated acting on the undergraduate question at the 1971 Annual Meeting. The fall 1970 minutes also include AUPHA's estimate that there were now approximately 20 operational bachelor-level programs.

July 1, 1970, was the federal deadline for practicing nursing home administrators to have secured their state licenses. While each state had different requirements, many demanded either an associate's degree or bachelor's degree as one qualification for licensure. Therefore, at approximately the same time that professional nursing home managers were striving to meet specific educational requirements, AUPHA had agreed to consider bachelor-level health administration programs for membership.

Minutes of the April 1970 AUPHA Annual Meeting indicate "undergraduate attendees" from Clemson University, Ithaca College, The Pennsylvania State University, and the University of Cincinnati. Interestingly, none of the undergraduate program directors who attended the 1969 AUPHA Annual Meeting returned in 1970. At the 1970 meeting, the AUPHA Curriculum Task Force on Long-Term Care discussed state licensure with a working group organized by the Public Health Service to advise the American Association of Junior Colleges (AAJC) in efforts to involve community colleges in activation of *health administration* education. By this time, AUPHA had secured Kellogg funding and staff and prioritized long-term care administration (Griffith, 1974). AHA and AUPHA joined this working group after AAJC sent a release to all of its members calling for the development of programs in "health care administration especially for persons interested in nursing homes and other long-term care facilities" (AUPHA Records, 1970c, p. 19).

The AUPHA Committee on Constitution and Bylaws also reported its recommendation involving "additional membership classes" at the April 1970 Annual Meeting (AUPHA Records, 1970b). The report mentioned the "sudden emergence and quick proliferation" of undergraduate programs in hospital administration and the "possibility that undergraduate programs could 'rapidly outnumber graduate programs.'" It questioned whether and how education programs for administrators of specialized health institutions (e.g., mental health facilities and nursing homes) should affiliate with AUPHA. It also mentioned the need for new membership categories to accommodate foreign academic programs and U.S. voluntary associations.

The AUPHA Committee on Constitution and Bylaws, chaired by Professor Gilbert Blain (Montreal), was convinced that the question of new membership categories and classes was bound to bring into discussion the very nature of AUPHA, its role and purposes, its scope, its relation with other higher education associations, and even its name. In hindsight, we must applaud Blain and this committee's insight. They also reported that they had met with the AUPHA Executive Committee in March 1970, and all agreed to postpone all constitutional changes in relation to new membership categories (AUPHA Records, 1970a).

Prior to the Annual Meeting, the AUPHA Executive Committee submitted its three questions for consideration by the membership:

1. Should the association adopt an active and supportive posture or passive posture toward the development of undergraduate programs?
2. Should this development proceed within the association or independently?
3. Should the association modify its structure to include undergraduate programs? (AUPHA Records, 1970c)

The Executive Committee's report also identified five factors favoring the modification of the AUPHA membership structure to accommodate undergraduate programs. They were as follows (AUPHA Records, 1970c):

1. Graduate and undergraduate programs moving forward together could benefit each other.
2. The field of health services administration must avoid fragmentation.
3. Graduate programs cannot and should not attempt to meet the vast unmet needs in our field.
4. There is common interest.
5. We need to organize for the benefit of the student.

The Executive Committee also indicated its concerns. First, the committee was worried about academic rigor and faculty quality. The official minutes state, "AUPHA has directed most of its recent efforts to upgrading and monitoring educational quality. The Accrediting Commission is the expression of that investment of energy. Bringing in undergraduate programs and encouraging them may dilute that effort" (AUPHA Records, 1970c, p. 33).

Its other concerns involved the potential number of undergraduate members. The committee's meeting minutes state the following:

> The control of the Association's efforts to upgrade graduate education may be lost by virtue of the sheer numbers of (undergraduate) programs, some of which may have different interests. There is also the question of our ability to retain our identity as [an] Association—[an] identity which is the result of considerable effort over two decades. (AUPHA Records 1970c, p. 33)

The April 1970 Annual Meeting was a critical milestone in the introduction of undergraduate programs into AUPHA. It demonstrated that association leadership understood the issues, perspectives, and ramifications and how they could affect the organization and the field. It also demonstrated AUPHA's willingness to evolve its mission and structure, and potentially accept undergraduate programs and the associated uncertainties.

The September 1970 minutes of the Executive Committee meeting document the continuing discussion of the undergraduate question and state plans for a January 1971 meeting with undergraduate faculty members (AUPHA Records, 1970c). At this time, there was no reason to believe that the Kellogg Foundation had changed its policy regarding its nonsupport for undergraduate programs.

1971: AUPHA's Plan for Baccalaureate Program Members

The January 1971 meeting of the Executive Committee reported AUPHA's plan for baccalaureate programs (AUPHA Records, 1971a). It proposed constitutional changes involving three membership categories: graduate, baccalaureate, and associate. ("Associate" in this context means an academic program that awards an associate's degree.) The meeting minutes stated that "Institutions desiring (baccalaureate) membership must agree to participate in peer review and that peer review must *not be interpreted as accreditation*" (emphasis added). AUPHA also mandated that undergraduate programs joining the association before the criteria for full voting membership are established would be admitted as associate (nonvoting) members (AUPHA Records, 1971a, pp. 1–2).

The minutes of the April 1971 AUPHA Annual Meeting report a lively debate on the undergraduate question and a proposed constitutional amendment to modify AUPHA's membership categories to include baccalaureate programs (AUPHA Records, 1971b). The proposed amendment was introduced *for discussion only*. No vote was taken. The discussion addressed many of the issues covered in this chapter. Professor Stephen Schneeweiss (Ithaca), Professor John MacLearn (Quinnipiac), Zacheus Okediji (Meherry Medical/Tennessee State University), and Professor George Wren (Georgia State) addressed many specific questions involving the need and demand for undergraduates with a degree in health administration and the articulation of undergraduate and graduate programs. Professor Marshall Raffel (Penn State) provided the central points of discussion for this meeting. He noted six relevant points that merited consideration (AUPHA Records, 1971c):

1. There is a need for continuing dialog between the undergraduate and graduate programs.
2. The number of undergraduate programs is growing, and they are a permanent fixture on the scene.
3. AUPHA is the logical locus for this dialogue.
4. Allied health is not a logical locus because the only thing administration has in common with allied health professionals is perhaps the word "health."
5. The American Public Health Association is not a logical locus because it is just too large.
6. A separate organization for undergraduate programs would simply divide the two groups.

Raffel's points served to focus the discussion along with the issues raised by Professors Hartman (Iowa), Dowling (Michigan), Dornblasser (Minnesota), and

Battistella (Cornell). Collectively, these discussions expressed the rationale for AUPHA to affiliate with undergraduate programs in *the name of mutual interest.* In spite of the angst and uncertainties associated with the undergraduate question, Raffel was able to present a positive, workable framework and rationale for an effective union between the two types of programs. While he acknowledged issues, his vision of an effective working union was clear.

The minutes of the August 1971 Executive Session at an AUPHA Interim Meeting include the AUPHA Executive Committee's specific recommendations concerning constitutional changes (AUPHA Records, 1971c). Members discussed the motion prior to a formal vote by AUPHA member programs. Since no undergraduate programs were full AUPHA members, they could not participate. The following is a comprehensive report of this discussion as reflected in the record. It demonstrates both support and opposition. It also demonstrates the serious consideration AUPHA member (graduate) programs gave to the undergraduate question.

- Professor Austin (Xavier) indicated his program's opposition to the motion to involve adding baccalaureate-level programs. He reported "fundamental doubts" as to the appropriateness of undergraduate education.
- Professor Thompson (Yale) also voiced opposition based on the ambiguity of undergraduate program goals and the negative implications of bringing undergraduate programs into AUPHA before they "legitimized their role" and before that role was in fact determined.
- Professor Stimson (California, Berkeley) also opposed the motion based on the vagueness of the criteria for membership.
- Professor Hamilt (Temple) indicated his faculty support for the inclusion of undergraduate members. He stated that "making believe that undergraduate programs do not exist, or closing the club to their membership can certainly have no positive impact."
- At this point in the discussion, Dowling offered an amendment to the original motion that clarified and expanded the required qualifications of the one faculty member required for baccalaureate-level membership. This motion addressed many of the concerns expressed by AUPHA membership. His motion to amend also mentioned that additional criteria for admission into AUPHA for full membership would be subject to ratification by the entire membership at a regular meeting. When the question was called, the motion to amend proposed by Dowling passed on a roll call vote.
- When discussion continued, Thompson raised the question of the coexistence of an undergraduate and graduate program on the same campus. He also brought up the issue that a university's graduate program

may not be accredited and therefore not be eligible for full AUPHA membership, while its undergraduate program on the same campus—in the absence of a formal accreditation requirement—could become a full AUPHA member.

- Professor Kroeger (Pittsburgh) observed that since accreditation was required to be a full member at the graduate level, it "would be easier" to become a full member at the baccalaureate level.
- Professor Galligher (Trinity) asked whether full member undergraduate programs would be eligible to vote on applications for graduate membership in the association. He was told yes.
- Professor Burnett (Tulane) also voiced concern regarding accreditation.
- Professor Kralewski (Colorado) indicated the association needed additional information before it could take any action.
- Professor Stephan (Minnesota) expressed concern about the effect inclusion of baccalaureate-level programs would have on AUPHA's relationships with the ACHA and their membership requirements.

The motion to adopt the amendment as amended was called. It did not secure the required two-thirds majority—it needed one additional vote to pass.

Even though it did not pass, the vote demonstrated the positive endorsement from a majority of the graduate program membership.

The November 1971 Executive Committee Meeting minutes indicate that the undergraduate question remained a viable topic and was again discussed. The Executive Committee interpreted the initial vote as a mandate to move ahead and find a solution to the undergraduate question. Even though some AUPHA leaders on the Executive Committee still doubted the desirability of adding undergraduate programs, under Dr. Filerman's guidance they worked to adhere to the will of the membership.

Several other substantive points were discussed at the November 1971 Executive Committee meeting. For example, there were revised criteria for withholding full undergraduate membership and voting privileges until the "undergraduate professional role is more fully described," and the criteria for *full* AUPHA undergraduate membership were developed to the satisfaction of the graduate programs. The committee also discussed revised plans, including barring admission of undergraduate programs to Associate Membership except upon application and review by the Executive Committee and approved by the majority of the membership. A significant change dropped the distinction between baccalaureate and associate degree levels and welcomed both levels of "undergraduate" programs into AUPHA. At this time, the Executive Committee also discussed changing its constitution and bylaws to include a new name for AUPHA.

1972: AUPHA's Plan B

In August 1972, Dr. Filerman sent a memo to the graduate program faculties to define two changes to its former proposal for undergraduate affiliation. First, AUPHA formally proposed changing its name, with one option being the Association of University Programs in Health Administration. Second, Dr. Filerman provided a revised proposal for undergraduate program membership—called Category B members—to all (graduate) member programs. This proposal dropped all references to "baccalaureate" level and instead included both baccalaureate and associate degree programs as "undergraduate" programs.

The memo identified the following potential baccalaureate program members:

1. Concordia (MN)
2. Georgia State
3. Ithaca College
4. The Pennsylvania State University

Potential associate degree members included

1. Essex Community College (MD),
2. Northwood Institute (MI),
3. St. Petersburg Junior College (FL), and
4. The State University, Agricultural and Technical College (Delhi, NY).

The modified amendment indicated that Category A (graduate full members) and Category B (undergraduate full members) would have equal vote "on the floor" at association meetings and that the majority of members on both the AUPHA executive and nominating committees would come from Category A members, with the minority drawn from Category B members. Therefore, the undergraduate question continued to mature and remain an open and high-priority debate for AUPHA's Executive Committee.

The minutes of the December 1972 Executive Committee Meeting indicate that the committee would formally propose changing the Hospital Administration portion of AUPHA's name to Health Administration. Those minutes also reflect that AUPHA received applications for associate (nonvoting) membership from Ithaca College and The George Washington University/U.S. Navy. The committee decided it would recommend these programs to the AUPHA membership at the 1973 Annual Meeting as "associate (non-voting) members" of AUPHA. These were the first membership applications received from undergraduate programs.

1973: Additional Applications for Associate Membership

The January 1973 Executive Committee minutes stated that AUPHA received applications for associate membership from the Northwood Institute and The Pennsylvania State University. Even though AUPHA had not yet approved the proposed Category B Membership, the association began accepting applications from undergraduate programs for associate (nonvoting) membership. The January 1973 meeting minutes also include some additional technical changes to the motion to change AUPHA's name and establish "undergraduate and other" membership categories. AUPHA sent informational copies of the revisions to all known undergraduate programs.

1974–1975: Eight Baccalaureate Programs Earn Full Membership

The AUPHA Executive Committee's minutes for April 1975 include the revised membership criteria for full (voting) undergraduate program membership. AUPHA membership accepted and approved these proposed changes. The minutes also indicate that eight undergraduate programs recommended by the "undergraduate steering committee" were peer reviewed using predetermined criteria and approved by the Executive Committee for Type B full membership. The eight were Ithaca College, Medical College of Virginia/Virginia Commonwealth University, The Pennsylvania State University, Providence College, Quinnipiac College, Sangamon State University, and Wichita State University.

Subsequent AUPHA minutes and reports reflect an increasing number of undergraduate associate and full members. By April 1977, AUPHA Board minutes reflect a functioning undergraduate presence in the association. Unfortunately, there was still some lingering tension, and the angst between undergraduate and graduate programs remained. At the April meeting, Professor Harold Cohen (Ithaca), AUPHA's first Board member from an undergraduate program, reported that the association needed to be more responsive in providing leadership and funding to undergraduate programs.

By the late 1970s and early 1980s, new leaders involved in the development of undergraduate programs emerged. Most noteworthy was Professor Carol J. Harten (Cincinnati), who succeeded Cohen on the AUPHA Board. She also chaired AUPHA's Undergraduate Task Force.

THE UNDERGRADUATE ERA: POST-1975

One can debate whether the "undergraduate era" began in 1973 when Ithaca College joined AUPHA as an associate member or when the original eight undergraduate programs earned full membership as Category B members. Because the original goal of the initiative was full voting membership, 1975 is a logical end point to the controversy and the dawn of a new era in which undergraduate programs were fully included in AUPHA.

Over time, undergraduate health administration education became a priority for AUPHA. It also eventually received significant support from the Kellogg Foundation. Undergraduate faculty joined AUPHA curriculum task forces, and these programs routinely met to continue refining their standards and accomplishments. AUPHA publications emerged, including *Baccalaureate Health Administration Graduates: A Decade Review* (Tourigny & LaFrance, 1983). In 1990, *Journal of Health Administration Education* published a special issue devoted to undergraduate education (Reagan, 1990).

LINGERING ISSUES AND CONCERNS

The process of bringing undergraduate programs into AUPHA created a number of issues. Whether they are significant or trivial today is a matter of perspective. For example, Dr. Filerman's editorial in the previously mentioned *Journal of Health Administration Education* special issue—published 15 years *after* undergraduate programs formally entered AUPHA—is especially noteworthy. In the article, he states, "Health services is a research-based field. Quality undergraduate education and health services research are inextricably linked. Institutions that do not encourage faculty research are not appropriate settings for health administration education." He goes on to write, "It is the time to close the era of undergraduate education as the retreat for faculty avoiding research" (Filerman, 1990, p. 159). This issue and concern were voiced earlier, as undergraduate education was being considered for inclusion in AUPHA. A search of association records reveals there has never been a systematic audit of the research productivity of undergraduate faculty. (Morrisey, Menachemi, Cawley, and Ginter [2010] provide an example of this type of audit for graduate faculty.) Then and today, AUPHA membership criteria have no formal expectations regarding faculty research productivity and do not require reporting of research activity.

In the first 15 years of undergraduate inclusion in AUPHA, membership criteria remained modest. This was a strategy to attract new and developing baccalaureate-level programs into AUPHA. Whether modest barriers of entry still reflected the best interests of our field and students remains a concern. Related to this is the apparent turnover of AUPHA's undergraduate membership, though factors of budget and reorganization are issues for some programs. For example, of the 53 undergraduate programs who joined AUPHA between 1973 and 1989, only 15 (28 percent) are still AUPHA members (Tourigny & LaFrance, 1983).

Another significant issue that remains involves the articulation between graduate and baccalaureate-level programs. Lee and Nowicki (2005) reported on the complexity of this issue. Until AUPHA addresses it systematically, baccalaureate and graduate programs remain related but independent, even if both exist in the same college or university. Whether this appropriately meets the needs of the field and its students remains unclear. Lee and Nowicki state, "The paper concludes that discussion of health administration degree articulation has received modest attention and discussion for more than twenty years, and neither formal relationships nor certification/accreditation has addressed the issue" (p. 221).

MOVING FORWARD

This chapter has chronicled how a reluctant AUPHA eventually folded undergraduate programs into its membership. It has called attention to early undergraduate faculty heroes and pioneers, most notably Professor Marshall Raffel (The Pennsylvania State University) and Professor Stephan Schneeweiss (Ithaca College). Other faculty, including Professors William Dowling and John Griffith (Michigan) and Milton Hamilt (Temple), provided significant input at critical times. The questions and issues expressed by Professor John Thompson (Yale) predicted many of the lingering issues still affecting baccalaureate programs today.

This chapter has also called attention to the wisdom of Dr. Filerman, who set the bar high so that if the undergraduate/AUPHA union was to occur, all participants could be winners in both the short and long term. Later chapters highlight his continuing leadership, including securing Kellogg Foundation funding to help baccalaureate programs mature in AUPHA.

While this chapter aims to reflect the events leading up to undergraduate program membership in AUPHA, the reader should not regard it to be a definitive history of undergraduate education over the last 40 to 50 years. That said, since affiliating with AUPHA, undergraduate health administration programs have matured and prospered. Raffel's original argument that working with undergraduate programs inside the AUPHA framework would benefit our field and students, although presenting substantial challenges, seems prophetic.

REFERENCES

AUPHA Records. (1968a). *AUPHA Executive Committee Minutes and Records*, September. Washington, DC: Association of University Programs in Health Administration.

AUPHA Records. (1968b). *AUPHA Executive Committee Minutes and Records*, December. Washington, DC: Association of University Programs in Health Administration.

AUPHA Records. (1970a). *AUPHA Executive Committee Minutes and Records*, March. Washington, DC: Association of University Programs in Health Administration.

AUPHA Records. (1970b). *AUPHA Executive Committee Minutes and Records*, April. Washington, DC: Association of University Programs in Health Administration.

AUPHA Records. (1970c). *AUPHA Executive Committee Minutes and Records*, September. Washington, DC: Association of University Programs in Health Administration.

AUPHA Records. (1971a). *AUPHA Executive Committee Minutes and Records*, January. Washington, DC: Association of University Programs in Health Administration.

AUPHA Records. (1971b). *AUPHA Executive Committee Minutes and Records*, April. Washington, DC: Association of University Programs in Health Administration.

AUPHA Records. (1971c). *AUPHA Executive Committee Minutes and Records*, August. Washington, DC: Association of University Programs in Health Administration.

Cohen, H. E. (1977). Baccalaureate education in health care administration. In J. P. Dixon (Ed.), *The report of the commission on education for health administration education, Volume III* (pp. 57–78). Ann Arbor, MI: Health Administration Press.

Filerman, G. L. (1983). An oral history. In L. E. Weeks (Ed.), *Hospital administration oral history collection*. Chicago, IL: Library of the American Hospital Association, Asa S. Bacon Memorial, and American Hospital Association.

Filerman, G. L. (1990). Editorial: Undergraduate professional education: Accomplishments and agenda (Special issue). *Journal of Health Administration Education*, *8*(2), 159–160.

Gordon, S. M. (1975). Relevance for what? Health programs in search of a goal. Paper presented at Program Director's Workshop. Bethesda, MD: Health Resources Administration.

Griffith, J. R. (1974). Guest editorial: Education for the profession—an AUPHA update. *Journal of Long Term Care Administration*, *2*(3), 1–4.

Hill, D., & Raffel, M. (1977). *Health planning and administration: The Pennsylvania State University's Baccalaureate Program.* University Park, PA: Pennsylvania State University.

Lee, J. M., & Nowicki, M. (2005). Articulation of undergraduate and graduate education in health administration: Barriers and struggles. *Journal of Health Administration Education, 22*(2), 221–231.

Loebs, S. (2001). The continuing evolution of health management education. *Journal of Health Administration Education Supplement,* 33–50.

Morrisey, M. A., Menachemi, N., Cawley, J., & Ginter, P. M. (2010). Publication activity of health administration faculty. *Journal of Health Administration Education, 27*(3), 199–217.

Reagan, J. T. (1990). Special issue: Undergraduate education in health administration. *Journal of Health Administration Education, 8*(2).

Schneeweiss, S. M. (1973). *Undergraduate education in health care administration: The Ithaca College experience: 1968–1973.* Ithaca, NY: Ithaca College.

Tourigny, A. W., & LaFrance, S. V. (1983). *Baccalaureate health administration graduates: A decade review.* Arlington, VA: AUPHA.

ABOUT THE AUTHOR

Lee F. Seidel, PhD, is Professor Emeritus of Health Management and Policy at the University of New Hampshire. He has been involved in undergraduate health administration education since 1977. For the last 24 years, he also has been a Visiting Professor with the Executive MBA Program in Health Administration at the University of Colorado, Denver. He was elected to the AUPHA Board in 1981 and was its first chair from a baccalaureate-level program from 1984 to 1985. Prior to his academic career, he was affiliated with Arthur Andersen and Company and the Office of the Mayor, City of New York.

CHAPTER 4

Improving Health Administration Education: The Evolution and Current Practice of Peer Evaluation and Standard Setting

Sherril B. Gelmon, DrPH, FACHE,
Margaret F. Schulte, DBA, FACHE, CPHIMS, and
Leigh W. Cellucci, PhD

INTRODUCTION

Throughout the history of health administration education, there has been a commitment to continuously improving program content, delivery, and style to respond to new trends in higher education and employers' changing needs. Currently in health administration education, peer review and the evaluation against predefined standards takes many forms, including accreditation for graduate programs, certification for undergraduate programs, and no consistent external peer review process for doctoral programs.

In this chapter, we will explore the evolution of these different approaches, identify key factors that have led to the current situation, and discuss options for the future.

ACCREDITATION: A BRIEF BACKGROUND

To begin this discussion, we focus on the core issue of the continuous improvement of the educational process and the preparation of graduates for the settings, contexts, and roles in which they will work. Standards are a core part of this effort, as is peer evaluation and professional input, but the key concept with which to begin is improvement. The focus on evaluation and improvement has grown in recent decades. Reasons for this growth include greater consumer advocacy and expectations of accountability, increased demand for resources and simultaneous constraints on availability, and expectations for higher education institutions to be increasingly responsive to community needs and integral engines of community development (Gelmon, 1995).

The process of peer review and evaluation against standards is often viewed as a regulatory, bureaucratic, potentially punitive, and time-consuming activity—not one that engenders enthusiasm or positive response. Yet this endeavor—whether formal accreditation, certification, or other standardized review—is intended to assure the public of educational program quality and relevance, while promoting continual examination and self-improvement by educational programs (Dickey, 1985; Filerman, 1984; Gelmon, O'Neil, Kimmey, & Task Force, 1999; Greene, 1984).

Educational accreditation and review in the United States operates as a nongovernmental, voluntary process with guided self-evaluation and improvement central to the activity. Specialized accreditation is both a process that entails the assessment of program quality and the continued enhancement of program operations, and a condition that provides a credential to the public that clearly states that a program fulfills its commitment to educational quality (ASPA, 1993).

U.S. accreditation programs for higher education are guided by program-specific sets of standards developed by independent organizations of academics, practitioners, and public representatives. They include a common set of components that address self-study, documentation preparation, on-site peer evaluation against standards, presentation of findings in a structured report, decision-making regarding accreditation status, and ongoing periodic review, updates, and reporting (ASPA, 2017; CHEA, 2017; Gelmon, 1995; Young, Chambers, Kells, & Associates, 1983).

Accreditation (and comparable forms of peer review) emerged in U.S. higher education as a response to questions about the quality of educational offerings, spurred by the 1862 Land Grant Act, which gave federal lands to states to establish state universities (Gelmon et al., 1999). The earliest health profession accreditation organizations emerged in the early 20th century (for example, medicine in 1904 and nursing in 1916) (Blauch, 1959). The 1910 Flexner Report on medical education resulted in new standards (Kells, 1994) and had a ripple effect across many professional education programs, resulting in increased scrutiny.

Throughout the late 19th and most of the 20th centuries, six regional accreditation associations evolved to improve relationships between secondary and higher education and strengthen college admissions standards. These associations focus at the institutional level. As the workforce has become increasingly professionalized and specialized, multiple academic programs have been developed to educate these new professionals, and specialized accrediting organizations have been established with profession-specific standards and evaluation programs (Gelmon et al., 1999). These independent associations are nongovernmental and have reinforced the "voluntary" nature of accreditation, in particular in nonlicensed professions such as health management.

Originally, health professions program accreditation was intended to achieve the goal of defining and meeting explicit standards that would protect the public's health, as well as the futures of students seeking education. Over time, accreditation has come to be viewed by some as recognition of a minimum threshold of quality, ensuring that no harm will come to a student enrolled in the approved program or to a patient or client served by a graduate of such a program. Throughout the late 20th century and into the recent past, both institutional and specialized accreditation were increasingly tied to government funding, eligibility for financial aid, and workforce regulation, compromising their "voluntary" nature. In response, there have been calls to rethink accreditation (Gelmon et al., 1999) and view it as a mechanism for the continuous improvement of higher education, which in turn, in the health professions, will affect health services delivery and the health of populations.

THE HISTORY OF HEALTH ADMINISTRATION GRADUATE PROGRAM ACCREDITATION

During the 1960s, AUPHA began to consider establishing an accreditation function to address the growing numbers of programs in what was then hospital administration. The field had grown relatively quickly following World War II and the Korean War, when veterans returned and sought to use their military leadership and battleground medical experience to find careers in healthcare. They were supported by the Servicemen's Readjustment Act (the GI Bill), and later by passage of similar legislation to support Vietnam veterans as they returned home.

This was also the era of a hospital building "boom" and the expansion of healthcare financial coverage. Financing grew through private insurance and with the passage of Medicare and Medicaid programs. People from all income strata and geographic areas quickly gained access to healthcare. With support from the W.K. Kellogg Foundation, early programs in hospital administration developed in schools of public health and other academic settings. For these programs to access federal funding, they needed to be accredited by a body that was recognized by the (then) U.S. Commissioner of Education in the Office of Education. The policy intent behind this requirement was to ensure program quality and integrity and prevent program proliferation. For AUPHA's member programs to participate, an accrediting body would need to be founded, launched, and then seek the recognition of the U.S. Commissioner of Education (Weeks, 1984).

The accreditation of health administration graduate programs began in 1968 with the establishment of the Accrediting Commission on Graduate Education for Hospital Administration (ACGEHA). AUPHA reached out to the field to gain the participation of professional and industry associations that represented the wide-ranging market for hospital administrators. ACGEHA was originally constituted with four corporate sponsors:

- The Association of University Programs in Health Administration
- The American College of Hospital Administrators
- The American Hospital Association
- The American Public Health Association

These sponsors represented the major stakeholders related to education and practice (both organizational and individual membership associations). In the mid-1970s, two public members were added as voting members of the commission (Gelmon, 1995).

In 1970, ACGEHA was officially recognized by the U.S. Office of Education, which served as a gatekeeper for federal funding to higher education. This recognition allowed ACGEHA-accredited programs to participate in federal student aid programs.

In 1975, ACGEHA changed its name to the Accrediting Commission on Education for Health Services Administration (ACEHSA) to reaffirm and reflect inclusion of the broader "health services" marketplace. While AUPHA's focus continued to remain primarily on hospitals, it, along with ACEHSA, recognized the broader, but fragmented, delivery continuum and range of financing organizations that served society's medical and health needs.

Over the next 30 years, additional organizations participated in ACEHSA. These corporate sponsors represented long-term care, health planning, mental health, medical practice, and Canadian health administrators.

The relevant governmental (U.S. Department of Education) and nongovernmental agencies (Council on Postsecondary Accreditation until 1993; Council for Higher Education Accreditation from 1993 to present) have continuously recognized ACGEHA and its successor organizations (ACEHSA and CAHME) since 1996.

As with other specialized accreditors, the primary functions of accreditation are to promote quality education by establishing criteria for the peer review of educational programs, conduct reviews of programs to determine compliance with these criteria, promote continuous self-improvement within the programs, and serve the public interest.

HISTORY OF HEALTH ADMINISTRATION UNDERGRADUATE PROGRAM CERTIFICATION

Baccalaureate programs in health administration date to the 1920s (AUPHA Task Force, 1978). In fact, the first undergraduate program was established at Marquette University in the late 1920s, while the first enduring graduate program was initiated at the University of Chicago in 1934 (Gelmon, 1990). Undergraduate programs first joined AUPHA in 1973, and over the years the requirements for program membership evolved (see Chapter 3). The W.K. Kellogg Foundation generously supported AUPHA from 1974 to 1990 to strengthen undergraduate program development, offer consultation to developing programs, and establish quality standards agreed upon by peers and monitored by AUPHA (Gelmon, 1990).

A substantive undergraduate membership panel review process was launched as a pilot in 1984 to respond to concerns that a self-study membership application might have questions about reliability and validity. This action also recognized that programs could not afford the costs of on-campus site visits associated with accreditation and other external review organizations. The panel review process was institutionalized in 1986 and continues (with refinements) to this day as the AUPHA undergraduate certification process (described in detail on the AUPHA [2017] website at http://www.aupha.org/main/membership/certification).

High academic standards form the foundation for certification review so that students who graduate from AUPHA-certified undergraduate programs enter the health management industry academically and professionally prepared for their careers. In early reviews, undergraduate curricula mirrored courses that were taught in master's-level programs to ensure student success (M. Nowicki, personal communication, June 5, 2017). Lloyd Burton, Professor Emeritus at Weber State University, stated:

> There was an evolution for the certification process that followed graduate program evolution. As they [graduate programs] adopted competency models, undergraduate programs began to look seriously at them as well. AUPHA review guidelines now include that they [undergraduate programs] must have a set of competencies to serve as curriculum foundation. (L. Burton, personal communication, June 8, 2017)

Including fieldwork experience as a program requirement allowed for deeper student evaluations as well as program improvements. Directors helped students develop and master communication and leadership competencies, and programs used fieldwork to assess student mastery of identified competencies. Fieldwork also provided outcomes data (via student self-assessment, preceptor evaluations, and faculty internship coordinator input) for curriculum revision to improve students' educational experiences and competency mastery (Thompson, 2005). Sasnett, Watkins, and Ferlazzo (2017) offer an example of students who worked as facilitators for patient-centered medical home recognition. Student self-assessment and preceptor and faculty internship coordinator evaluations noted student competency development in leadership, teamwork, and communication. The fieldwork experience (introduced when AUPHA membership guidelines were established) continues to be a valid pedagogy for student success and illustrates the value of AUPHA requirements for program excellence.

Academic standards were a key foundational element when undergraduate membership requirements were adopted by AUPHA in 1975, and eight programs became members. This number has since grown to 87 undergraduate members in 2017. The emphasis on standards was a significant factor in spurring continued growth in the number of programs interested in maintaining high-quality education recognized by an outside certifying body (AUPHA). Table 4.1 illustrates the growth in undergraduate AUPHA membership from 1990 to the present (C. Sanyer, personal communication, June 21, 2017; Gelmon, 1990).

The AUPHA Undergraduate Program Committee has regularly revisited the certification criteria, revising them to reflect changes in policy, technology, and industry. Nonetheless, the certification process remains similar to the original process adopted in 1984 (C. Sanyer, personal communication, June 21, 2017; Gelmon, 1990). The underlying driver for certification and program requirements is to meet or exceed AUPHA-defined academic standards.

In addition to meeting eligibility requirements regarding governance, faculty expertise, and curriculum, programs prepare a self-study that reviews program structure, faculty, and resources; student support services; linkages with professionals and alumni; and curriculum structure and content that includes examples of experimental and applied learning. Programs provide evidence of program evaluation and improvement regarding the assessment of student learning and programmatic outcomes.

Table 4.1. AUPHA Undergraduate Program Membership

Status	1990	2000	2010	2017
Full certification	26	21	45	45
Associate member	7	13	22	42
Total	33	34	67	87

Throughout the 30 years of AUPHA undergraduate program review and certification, a number of themes have emerged that distinguish yet complement the certification process as compared to the graduate accreditation process. The journey toward certification, while rigorous, has generally been collegial. Carla Wiggins, Professor at Weber State University, noted, "It was a process of user-friendly program building" (C. Wiggins, personal communication, June 11, 2017). John Seavey, Professor Emeritus at the University of New Hampshire and former AUPHA Board Chair, described program reviews as follows: "We sought to be encouraging and give a lot of feedback to improve their programs . . . the process was academics talking with academics who work for program improvement" (J. Seavey, personal communication, June 21, 2017).

This philosophy of mentoring, collegiality, and camaraderie was ever-present and emphasized in AUPHA trainings and in curricular and website documents. AUPHA created the places and spaces for undergraduate faculty to engage in the positive exchange of ideas. The *Journal of Health Administration Education* has published articles and cases relevant to undergraduate education, and two special issues have been dedicated to the topic (in 1990 and 2005). AUPHA Annual Meetings now include an undergraduate program breakfast that guarantees a dedicated time and place for undergraduate faculty to meet and discuss program issues. The Undergraduate Program Workshops (held every two years) are built around a theme of interest for program and faculty development. These workshops provide networking opportunities, promote the exchange of ideas for curriculum and program improvement, and facilitate research team-building. As one key informant observed, "The Undergraduate Program Workshops made us feel we had an important part of AUPHA. Our [undergraduate] degree had value" (L. Rubino, personal communication, June 5, 2017).

In addition, AUPHA's Faculty Forums offer undergraduate program faculty a place to exchange ideas and build knowledge with graduate faculty on topic areas relevant to program development. The current use of online forums facilitates this exchange and builds a shared philosophy of mentoring, collegiality, and camaraderie without regard to undergraduate or graduate status. Faculty and AUPHA have partnered on the common theme of academic standards and excellence in education.

ACCREDITATION'S EMPHASIS AND FOCUS

During the 1970s and 1980s, accreditation criteria reflected the field of the time. The small but specialized interconnected groups of faculty in the core disciplines, such as social sciences, management functions, quantitative methods, law, and so on, guided criteria and process development (S. Sundre, personal communication, May 13, 2017). Criteria also reflected the influence of the predominance of schools of public health in which many programs were situated.

During the 1980s, ACEHSA was the stable, but small, accrediting organization that accredited several dozen graduate programs (S. Sundre, personal communication, May 13, 2017). When the focus on cost containment intensified during the late 1980s and into the 1990s, health services delivery evolved and new payment models (particularly the adoption of the prospective payment system and the Diagnostic Related Groups payment model) drove a focus on outcomes measurement and fostered a growing competitive environment for healthcare services. The shift to ambulatory surgical and diagnostic services, and consolidation of providers along the care continuum, intensified with a focus on provider integration within single organizational structures. Competition among what were previously separate but collegial provider organizations became fierce as each positioned for market share.

Surviving and thriving in this new competitive environment called for skills that healthcare leaders had not honed over the prior decades. Strategic thinking and managing diverse resources along the care continuum, developing innovative financial strategies, and managing accountability based on measurable clinical and financial performance outcomes were paramount. The changing demands called for competencies that had not previously been the focus of healthcare leaders' professional development or graduate education.

While healthcare was changing rapidly, higher education was also exploding with the development of nontraditional (i.e., part-time) programs, distance education, and the continuously growing market for management talent in all healthcare segments. As the focus on outcomes measurement evolved in health services with measurable results assessed using clinical data, there were no adequate competency frameworks, evaluation standards, or assessment models. Higher education lacked the tools for measurement (S. Sundre, personal communication, May 13, 2017).

With AUPHA's leadership, ACEHSA began developing niche content areas that had not previously been the focus of curricula but that were in demand, such as process and quality improvement, information management, and outcomes assessment, resulting in the creation of various curriculum resources intended to assist programs in addressing these areas (see, for example, Austin & Pew Information Management Task Force, 1990; Dornblaser & Shalowitz, 1995; Gelmon, Baker, Evans, & Gustafson, 1994; Gelmon & Reagan, 1995). Accreditation standards evolved with increasing emphasis on niche curricula areas and included requirements for content that addressed related domains.

In 1988, ACEHSA embarked on a major review of its accreditation criteria, policies, and procedures, seeking to reflect advances in knowledge and practice and ensure that accreditation judgments remained objective and consistent (Gelmon,

O'Brien, Conrad, & Shortell, 1990a). This review was guided by a set of working assumptions designed to shape the future of ACEHSA's practice:

- Quality assurance and enhancement
- Affirmation of the role of ACEHSA
- Definition of the health services administration field
- Relative emphasis on structure, process, and outcomes
- Prescriptive versus flexible accreditation criteria
- Durability of criteria
- Market assumptions
- Curriculum content relevance
- Role of field work

The resulting revised 1990 *Criteria for Accreditation* and related policies reflected extensive consultations with the field through presentations, written comments, and open meetings. Of note at the time, there were multiple Canadian programs accredited by ACEHSA, and the Commission pursued a parallel strategy of consultation with Canadian educators and practitioners to ensure their input (Gelmon, O'Brien, Conrad, & Shortell, 1990b).

EVOLUTION TO COMMISSION ON ACCREDITATION OF HEALTHCARE MANAGEMENT EDUCATION

As healthcare became more complex and mergers and expansions led to ever-larger delivery enterprises, the demand for leadership competencies shifted again (S. Hernandez, personal communication, June 13, 2017). While AUPHA and ACEHSA began addressing and integrating the concept of improvement through the Pew Task Force on Quality Improvement (1990–1992), collaborations with the Institute for Healthcare Improvement that began in 1991, and the ACEHSA review process (1988–1990), the focus among healthcare leaders turned more intensely to performance improvement with the publication of the Institute of Medicine reports *To Err Is Human* (Kohn, Corrigan, & Donaldson, 2000) and *Crossing the Quality Chasm* (Institute of Medicine, Committee on Quality of Health Care in America, 2001).

In this environment, health administration education came under the microscope. "Are the graduates of health administration programs competent and prepared to manage in today's more complex and dynamic health organizations? What is the role of accreditation in ensuring the competency of our graduates?" (Campbell & Hilberman, 2004, p. 108). These questions were on the minds of representatives from academic programs in health services administration and practitioner organizations in February 2001 when they came together during a summit meeting in Orlando, Florida.

The summit concluded with the appointment of the Blue Ribbon Task Force (BRTF), whose mission was to examine "the way in which graduate programs in health administration are accredited and to make recommendations about the process and content of future accreditation" (Leatt et al., 2004, p. 116). The summit action plan included a call for a clarified and broader field definition similar to the question that was addressed when ACEHSA changed its name to reflect the broader health services administration field back in the 1970s. The 2004 BRTF report, completed after nearly three years of work, called for a closer partnership between practice and academe to support higher education in recognizing and responding to market demands.

Among its many other recommendations, the BRTF called for ACEHSA to do the following (Leatt, 2004):

1. Recraft its vision, including a redefinition to recognize the breadth of the field beyond hospital administration
2. Adopt a broader definition of *health services administration*
3. Adopt a core set of competencies that all program graduates would be expected to have mastered by graduation
4. Commit to ongoing evaluation of educational outcomes, particularly in the core competencies
5. Adopt an enhanced commitment to ensure that accreditation criteria address continuous quality improvement
6. Streamline the accreditation process
7. Deepen practitioner involvement through expanded sponsorships
8. Clarify the relationship between AUPHA and ACEHSA

ACEHSA had been considering actions to achieve greater autonomy and independence since 1994 and moved quickly and thoughtfully to address the BRTF recommendations. Within a short time, it made several strategic changes. In 2004, for example, the organization had changed its name to the Commission on Accreditation of Healthcare Management Education (CAHME). This was done primarily to be inclusive of the broader health management field, recognize the need for leadership and management in the wide range of settings in which healthcare is delivered, and acknowledge the range of interests that directly influence healthcare, such as public policy and regulation.

In light of the BRTF report, the organizational structure of what became CAHME was redesigned to establish a corporate member framework that was meant to provide oversight to ensure that accredited programs respond to the demands of the field. This structure also appointed the CAHME Board of Directors. Corporate members were required to provide financial support for the commission through annual fees (S. Hernandez, personal communication, June 13, 2017). It adopted bylaws that specified that the Board of Directors would comprise equal members from academe, practice, and the profession. Additionally, the board was designed to include public members and the CAHME President/CEO. This structure was a departure from the ACEHSA organization in which the accreditation commissioners served as the board, established accreditation standards and criteria, and made accreditation determinations (J. Lloyd, personal communication, June 15, 2017). Under the new structure, two new councils—the Accreditation and Standards Councils—report to the Board of Directors. The Board of Directors, in turn, reports to the corporate members at their annual meeting. Only the Board of Directors is authorized to make accreditation decisions.

In a further significant move, CAHME was separated from the organizational structure of AUPHA through a clear division of staffing and financing. Although ACEHSA had been incorporated as a distinct legal entity, it shared office space with AUPHA and had a number of operational agreements. The corporation was renamed (to CAHME), separated all operational elements, and moved to its own offices. While CAHME continues to function in close affiliation with AUPHA, it no longer has operating agreements with the association. However, AUPHA continues to serve as one of CAHME's corporate members, with a key role of recommending academic representatives to the CAHME Board of Directors. Likewise, CAHME's president is invited to attend all AUPHA Board meetings.

CAHME—A Perspective on Our First 50 Years

Anthony C. Stanowski, DHA, FACHE, President and CEO of CAHME

The author Pearl Buck once wrote "the test of a civilization is the way that it cares for its helpless members" (Buck, 1954, p. 337).

Surely this is one of the motivating factors behind the development of modern healthcare. As healthcare continues to evolve, physicians, nurses, employees, donors, and volunteers affirm human dignity by helping those in need. To borrow the words engraved above an old entrance to Bryn Mawr Hospital (Pennsylvania), hospitals are "dedicated to the healing of the sick, to the comfort of the suffering, and to the conservation of the life in the community." It is a noble and honorable cause.

(continued)

Fifty years ago, a group of visionaries realized that nobility, honor, and good intentions were not enough. That is when leaders from the American Hospital Association, the American College of Hospital Administrators (the predecessor of the American College of Healthcare Executives, ACHE), the American Public Health Association, and AUPHA came together to form the Accrediting Commission on Education for Hospital Administration. Their goal was to advance graduate education in hospital management. "Hospital" was quickly changed to "Health Services," reflecting that graduates served a broader purpose than hospital management. Today, the Commission on Accreditation of Healthcare Management Education (after a name change in 2004) continues to meet the mission established at its founding on January 1, 1968: to advance the quality of graduate healthcare management education.

Fifty years ago, our founders worked to create a process for instilling the scientific method in graduate healthcare management education. Today, CAHME's standards serve to ensure that our graduates have the competencies to lead in an era of ceaseless change.

At the dawn of our organization, our founders recognized that processes of education would change, and so focused on measuring the outcomes that demonstrate that graduates of CAHME-accredited programs are well prepared. Today, while programs still provide on-site "residential" experiences for full-time students, our programs and accreditation standards have evolved to account for the needs of part-time students seeking to advance their careers and the rise of online learning. While the mode of delivery may change, CAHME's mission is not compromised; the stakes are too high.

While fulfilling our mission as an accreditor, we accomplish it as professionals. Scores of practitioners and academics volunteer their time as a community of scholars in the accreditation process. It is a working body, the "wisdom of the crowd," in which a variety of healthcare providers, suppliers, professionals, insurers, and academics share perspectives on their aspirations for the field.

What sets students from CAHME-accredited programs apart is the knowledge that healthcare is different from other business models. CAHME graduates learn how to lead within the constant change of healthcare. They learn that resources must be invested with efficiency to improve care delivery, and that principles of our common humanity cannot be compromised. CAHME graduates learn how to lead with compassion, with an understanding that our delivery of healthcare reflects who we are as a society and what we aspire to be. CAHME recognizes that there is a noble purpose and honor in leading a healthcare institution.

Like all human enterprises, however, healthcare sometimes reflects the shortfalls and failures inherent in the social, political, and economic fabric of nations. Still, CAHME graduates strive for the ideal, for social justice, for change that increases and improves service to communities across the nation. It is right that our graduates work to achieve these worthy goals. CAHME is the bedrock on which our graduates, our future leaders, learn what it means to lead in healthcare and in the community.

Another important outcome of the BRTF report was the transition over time to a competency-based accreditation framework. CAHME moved from accreditation criteria based on specific curriculum content requirements to an outcomes-focused approach (M. Stefl, personal communication, May 15, 2017). This new methodology requires that programs clarify their missions based on the professional health services delivery sectors that are relevant to their graduates, and design their curricula based on the competencies needed for leaders and managers in the defined sector(s). This reflects CAHME's "mission-driven" orientation, which enables programs to shape their offerings around their specific missions, rather than being expected to conform to a predefined mission set for all programs seeking accreditation.

The competency-based framework also requires that programs measure their students' acquisition of competencies to ensure that graduates are prepared for the leadership roles that they will encounter in their professional lives. This emphasis is not unique to CAHME, and in fact is being observed by most of the specialized accreditors. However, even though all of them emphasize competencies and outcomes, few have created clear direction or have role models to help programs attempting to reframe their curricula and measurement systems.

The federal funding programs for graduate students in health services management were discontinued in the late 1990s. However, CAHME continued to retain U.S. Department of Education (USDE) recognition until 2014, when the USDE narrowed its gatekeeping focus to agencies that accredit programs eligible for federal student aid under Title IV programs. CAHME programs no longer have access to this funding, and so recognition by USDE was no longer required. CAHME opted to withdraw from USDE recognition in late 2014 (E. Brichto, personal communication, September 20, 2017).

CAHME gained and maintains recognition as the accrediting body for graduate programs in health management by the Council for Higher Education Accreditation (CHEA). CHEA represents approximately 3,000 academic institutions throughout the country and is the only nongovernmental body that recognizes—through a rigorous process of scrutiny and affirmation—the quality of accrediting bodies in the United States.

CAHME is also part of a broader community of specialized accreditors. ACEHSA was a founding member of the Association of Specialized and Professional Accreditors (ASPA), and its then–executive director was the founding chair of ASPA. ACEHSA, and subsequently CAHME, have maintained currency with the specialized accrediting community through ASPA membership and participation, accessing professional development for accreditation staff and participating in policy development relevant to the broader networks of specialized and professional accreditors.

UNDERGRADUATE CERTIFICATION TODAY AND GOING FORWARD

When AUPHA certifies or recertifies an undergraduate program, it communicates that this program embodies excellence and innovation in health services management education. The status of full certification is the "hallmark of quality" (Benson & Thompson, 2014).

One concern for the undergraduate programs, which is also relevant for the graduate programs, is the competition for resources. AUPHA undergraduate programs are housed in multiple academic units, such as the schools of business, public health, and liberal arts and sciences. Health management programs may prosper within these structures; however, they must be able to demonstrate the value added by AUPHA undergraduate membership (and program certification), especially for programs that coexist in an environment with other recognition/accreditation oversight. An undergraduate health administration program located in a business school might be included in a school-level accreditation by the Association to Advance Collegiate Schools of Business, the primary business school accreditor. Similarly, a program in a school of public health might be included in accreditation granted by the Council on Education for Public Health. It is incumbent upon the health administration program to demonstrate how AUPHA recognition and membership enhance the program's reputation.

Given the presence of competency or certification examinations in many disciplines, AUPHA's Undergraduate Program Committee has recommended the association consider establishing a comprehensive undergraduate end-of-program exit examination. The results could be used to provide feedback to students on their mastery of competencies and course material, provide information for program improvements, and offer graduating students from AUPHA undergraduate programs a recognition of excellence.

Another issue for continuing consideration is the establishment of articulation agreements with CAHME-accredited graduate programs. There is the potential that students who graduate from a certified AUPHA program would have benefits (such as advanced placement) if they pursue graduate education in health management.

A concern for both undergraduate and graduate programs is the assurance of quality and program integrity for online programs. While there is confidence in the quality assurance processes of certification and accreditation when reviewing traditional on-campus, face-to-face instruction, there is concern regarding how online programs meet student needs and maintain program excellence. These concerns center on examination proctoring, internship placements and supervision, and professional development opportunities.

Student mastery of cultural and diversity competencies in response to the need for a well-prepared, culturally diverse health administration workforce are critical for both undergraduate and graduate programs. Continued discussion of how programs may better address this is a focus for both the AUPHA Undergraduate Committee and CAHME. As one key informant stated, "We just need our graduates to better reflect the communities in which we live. This starts with undergraduate programs, and we have an opportunity to make a profound difference" (L. Friedman, personal communication, June 6, 2017).

LOOKING TO THE FUTURE

Following CAHME's transition from its long history as ACEHSA to a name and identity that reflects today's demands of healthcare leadership, the agency continues to refine and clarify the accreditation standards, as well as the criteria and related processes under which accreditation is provided. In the decade that has transpired since the adoption of a competency-based accreditation approach, health management graduate programs are slowly moving to adopt and adapt competency-based curricula and implement relevant teaching and assessment methods. The results of these efforts are yet to be measured in terms of their impacts on graduates' preparedness for their leadership and management roles.

In the context of undergraduate education, issues that were identified in 1990 for the coming decade (Seavey, 1990) continue to be relevant in 2017: a liberal education that complements preparation for a health administration career, education of generalists versus specialists, the centrality of management theory and practice, linkages with the health services industry, reliance upon faculty with expertise in the various disciplines of health administration, curriculum articulation, and peer review.

In terms of both undergraduate and graduate education, there will be continuing challenges to respond to the changing expectations of postmillennial students while adapting to new technologies and evolving education delivery modes. The health services delivery environment is also evolving, and new career opportunities are presented by both delivery sites and financing modes. Curricula will need to be adapted to respond to these opportunities, and faculty will need to stay current with the expectations of employers and other stakeholders.

The processes of peer review, standard setting, and quality assurance in health administration education will remain sensitive to what is expected by the practice community, and what practitioners expect of academic programs and their graduates. Continued confusion over the "turf" of health administration education will only be resolved as programs clarify their "domains" of knowledge, skills, abilities, and expertise with respect to educators in business, public health, public administration and policy, systems science, health informatics, and related social sciences.

The future of peer review in education rests in continued vigilance to maintain a system based on stakeholder expectations, competency definitions for graduates that are in alignment with practice and relevant to the level of the learner, independence and objectivity in the review system, and decision-making clarity and continuity. AUPHA, in collaboration with key stakeholders, has played a major role in peer review throughout its history. It should continue to be a key partner in the successful preparation of new members of the health administration professional workforce.

REFERENCES

Association of Specialized and Professional Accreditors. (1993). *The role and value of specialized accreditation: A policy statement*. Arlington, VA: Author.

Association of Specialized and Professional Accreditors. (2017). About accreditation. Retrieved from http://www.aspa-usa.org/about-accreditation/

Association of University Programs in Health Administration. (2017). Certification. Retrieved from http://www.aupha.org/main/membership/certification

AUPHA Task Force on Undergraduate Education. (1978). *An introduction to baccalaureate education for health administration*. Washington, DC: Association of University Programs in Health Administration.

Austin, C. J., & Pew Information Management Task Force. (1990). *Course content outlines for teaching information management in health administration*. Arlington, VA: Association of University Programs in Health Administration.

Benson, K., & Thompson, J. (2014). Charting a course to become AUPHA certified: What every undergraduate healthcare management program should know. *Journal of Health Administration Education, 31*(1), 75–84.

Blauch, L. E. (1959). *Accreditation in higher education.* Office of Education. Washington, DC: U.S. Government Printing Office.

Buck, P. S. (1954). *My several worlds.* (1st ed.). New York, NY: John Day Company.

Campbell, C., & Hilberman, D. (2004). Accreditation in health administration education: A call for change. *Journal of Health Administration Education, 21*(2), 107–114.

Council for Higher Education Accreditation. (2017). Information about accreditation. Retrieved from http://www.chea.org

Dickey, F. G. (1985). Accreditation in the allied health professions. In J. Hamburg (Ed.), *Review of allied health education,* 5 (pp. 107–125). Lexington, KY: University Press of Kentucky.

Dornblaser, B. M., & Shalowitz, J. I. (1995). Quality improvement in health management education (Special Issue). *Journal of Health Administration Education, 13*(Winter), 1–196.

Filerman, G. L. (1984). The influence of policy objectives on professional education and accreditation: The case of hospital accreditation. *Journal of Health Administration Education, 2*(Fall), 431–457.

Gelmon, S. B. (1990). Development of baccalaureate health administration education. *Journal of Health Administration Education, 8*(2), 227–244.

Gelmon, S. B. (1995). *Accreditation as a stimulus for continuous improvement in health management education: A case study of ACEHSA* (Doctoral dissertation, College of Healthcare Executives). Portland State University, Portland, OR.

Gelmon, S. B., Baker, G. R., Evans, J. P., & Gustafson, D. H. (1994). *A quality improvement teaching resource guide.* Arlington, VA: Association of University Programs in Health Administration and Institute for Healthcare Improvement.

Gelmon, S. B., O'Brien, D. M., Conrad, D. A., & Shortell, S. M. (1990a). Educating healthcare leaders for the 21st century: Evolution not revolution. *Healthcare Executive, 5*(January/February), 34–37.

Gelmon, S. B., O'Brien, D. M., Conrad, D. A., & Shortell, S. M. (1990b). Evolution not revolution: Health administration education for the 21st century. *Healthcare Management Forum, 3*(Spring), 25–29.

Gelmon, S. B., O'Neil, E. H., Kimmey, J. R., & the Task Force on Accreditation of Health Professions Education. (1999). *Strategies for change and improvement: The report of the task force on accreditation of health professions education*. San Francisco, CA: University of California, San Francisco.

Gelmon, S. B., & Reagan, J. T. (1995). *Assessment in a quality improvement framework: A sourcebook for health administration education*. Arlington, VA: Association of University Programs in Health Administration.

Greene, B. R. (1984). The context and role of specialized accreditation. *Journal of Health Administration Education, 2*(Fall), 409–418.

Institute of Medicine, Committee on Quality of Health Care in America. (2001). *Crossing the quality chasm: A new health system for the 21st century*. Washington, DC: National Academies Press.

Kells, H. R. (1994). *Self-study process: A guide for postsecondary and similar service-oriented institutions and programs*. Phoenix, AZ: American Council on Education and The Oryx Press.

Kohn, L. T., Corrigan, J. M., & Donaldson, M. S. (2000). *To err is human: Building a safer health system*. Washington, DC: National Academies Press.

Leatt, P. (2004). The continuous pursuit of quality through accreditation. *Journal of Health Administration Education, 21*(2), 115–120.

Leatt, P., Grady, R., Begun, J. W., Hernandez, S. R., Hilberman, D. W., Leach, D. C., . . . Sinioris, M. E. (2004). The final report of the Blue Ribbon Task Force on accreditation. *Journal of Health Administration Education, 21*(2), 121–166.

Sasnett, B., Watkins, R., & Ferlazzo, M. (2017). Health service management interns serve as practice facilitators for patient-centered medical home recognition. *The Health Care Manager, 36*(1), 96–103.

Seavey, J. W. (1990). Undergraduate health administration education in the 1990s. *Journal of Health Administration Education, 8*(Spring), 165–183.

Thompson, J. (2005). Competency development and assessment in undergraduate healthcare management programs: The role of internships. *Journal of Health Administration Education, 22*(4), 417–433.

Weeks, L. (Ed.). (1984). *Gary L. Filerman: In first person, An oral history*. Chicago, IL: American Hospital Association.

Young, K. E., Chambers, C. M., Kells, H. R., & Associates. (1983). *Understanding accreditation*. San Francisco, CA: Jossey-Bass Inc.

ABOUT THE AUTHORS

Sherril B. Gelmon, DrPH, FACHE, is Professor in the Oregon Health and Science University and Portland State University School of Public Health and directs the PhD Program in Health Systems and Policy. She teaches health systems management and policy in the graduate programs and leads multiple improvement science curricula for OHSU. Her research addresses improving health services delivery, health workforce development, and community engagement. She was Executive Director of ACEHSA and Director of Academic Affairs for AUPHA from 1988 to 1994. She received her doctorate in health policy from the University of Michigan; her master's in health administration from the University of Toronto; and undergraduate physiotherapy degrees from the Universities of Toronto and Saskatchewan.

Margaret F. Schulte, DBA, FACHE, CPHIMS (retired), is immediate past President and CEO of the Commission on Accreditation of Healthcare Management Education. Previously, she served on the faculty of the Northwestern University Masters of Science in Medical Informatics program; as Editor of *Frontiers in Health Services Management*, a publication of the American College of Healthcare Executives; and as Vice President of Education for the Healthcare Information and Management Systems Society. Previous positions were in healthcare association program management, academia, and healthcare management. She is a Fellow of the American College of Healthcare Executives.

Leigh W. Cellucci, PhD, is Associate Dean for Academic Affairs and Professor in the Department of Health Services and Information Management, College of Allied Health Sciences, East Carolina University. She has received the University of North Carolina Board of Governors Distinguished Professor for Teaching Award. Her research primarily centers on the strategic use of health information technology, examining factors that influence adoption and implementation of electronic health records, and has been published in journals such as *Health Policy and Technology*, *Business Case Journal*, and *Journal of Health Administration Education*. She is the author of three books focusing on healthcare management.

CHAPTER 5

Diversity in Health Management Education

Rupert M. Evans, DHA, FACHE,
Raymond Grady, MHA, FACHE, and
Diane M. Howard, PhD, FACHE

INTRODUCTION

Starting in 1968, major social forces and strong political leadership helped bring about the increase in minority enrollment in the health professions. At that time, the climate of the civil rights era and good economic times in the United States converged, and the nation seemed poised to commit itself to overcoming the barriers to full participation by minorities in health professions. The healthcare industry began to see more underrepresented minority individuals entering the workforce, and many health provider organizations continued to serve an increasingly diverse population, especially in major metropolitan communities. Leaders realized that increasing the healthcare workforce's racial and ethnic diversity was essential for the adequate provision of culturally competent care to burgeoning minority communities in the United States.

The consensus was that a diverse healthcare workforce would help expand healthcare access for underserved populations, focus research in neglected areas of societal need, and grow the pool of managers and policymakers to meet the needs of diverse populations. The long-term solution to achieving adequate diversity in the health professions depended on enhancing the diversity pipeline of health administration faculty and students. Affirmative action programs in health professions and healthcare management programs were critical to achieving a diverse healthcare workforce.

The journey toward increasing diversity in healthcare management education has not been without its challenges. While some progress has been made, there is plenty of room for improvement. Currently, African Americans, Hispanic Americans, and Native Americans constitute almost 30 percent of the U.S. population. However, in 2007, these groups accounted for only 9 percent of physicians, 7 percent of dentists, 10 percent of pharmacists, and 6 percent of registered nurses (Sullivan &

Mittman, 2010). Minority representation among academic faculty, deans, provosts, hospital administrators, and other health leadership positions is even more scant. During the 2007–2008 academic year, underrepresented minorities made up only 7 percent of total U.S. medical school faculty, less than 7 percent of undergraduate faculty, less than 10 percent of baccalaureate and graduate nursing school faculty, 12 percent of clinical psychology faculty, and 7 percent of dental school faculty (Sullivan & Mittman, 2010).

In 2008, Blacks and Hispanic Americans constituted 1 percent and 3 percent of full professors in medical schools, respectively, while they comprised 4 percent and 5 percent of associate professors. Native Americans and Native Hawaiians together constituted only 23 of 29,957 full medical school professors (0.08 percent) and 25 of 26,366 associate medical school professors (0.09 percent). These data were contained in the Sullivan Report (Sullivan & Mittman, 2010), which surveyed the presence of underrepresented minorities on medical, nursing, and dental school faculties. The Sullivan Report found that African Americans, Hispanics, and Native Americans were "missing." The report specifically addressed the pipeline to the healthcare professions and provided strategies to broaden this pipeline (Moore, Eder, & Dotson, 2013). It stated that diversity should be a core value in the health professions. Health professional schools should also ensure their mission statements reflect a social contract with the community and a commitment to diversity among their students, faculty, staff, and administration (Sullivan & Mittman, 2010). These data are well known to the Association of University Programs in Health Administration (AUPHA), and there has been a long-term strategic interest in diversifying the health management field.

THE EARLY WORK

A key moment in the evolution of diversity in healthcare management came in 1968 at the American Hospital Association (AHA) Annual Meeting in Atlantic City, New Jersey. Prior to the meeting, a number of African Americans in New York City, who held decision-making positions in medicine, nursing, and health management, had been networking in their respective workplaces about the paucity of Blacks and other minorities in the operation of professional institutions and organizations. During the AHA meeting, Whitney Young, president of the National Urban League, gave the keynote address, challenging hospitals to employ and promote minority leadership and administratively reflect the communities in which they resided (ACHE, 2008; Collins et al., 2008). These discussions about the opportunities that existed to expand efforts on behalf of minorities resulted in the formation of the National Association of Health Services Executives (NAHSE) during the AHA meeting. NAHSE's mission was—and continues to be—to advance and develop Black healthcare leaders and elevate the quality of healthcare services rendered to minority and underserved communities (ACHE, 2008). NAHSE established chapters around the country, with most organized in urban areas. The first, and most prominent, was in New York City, where NAHSE's founders worked and resided.

NAHSE was joined by several of AHA's Latino members in advocating for leadership opportunities in healthcare. These groups had a critical role in shaping the dialog with the American College of Healthcare Executives (ACHE), AHA, and AUPHA.

Haynes Rice—NAHSE national president from 1971 to 1973 and a healthcare executive at the New York City Health and Hospitals Corporation as well as a University of Chicago MBA graduate—formed an early relationship with then AUPHA president/CEO Gary Filerman, PhD (Weeks, 1984b), to further diversity in healthcare management education. In 1970, AUPHA and NAHSE collaborated on developing a summer work–study program with the goal of recruiting minority students to graduate programs (Collins et al., 2008). Up to that point, minority student enrollment in AUPHA graduate programs was very low. In 1967, it was less than 2 percent, and minority membership in ACHE was less than 1 percent. By 1969, both the number of minorities graduating from and those enrolling in AUPHA programs had fallen to less than 1 percent (Weeks, 1984b).

Dr. Filerman recruited Robert Detore to assume the director of student recruitment role. Mr. Detore had developed a minority healthcare careers program for Schering-Plough in 1968 in which 30 high school students were provided internships at various hospitals in the New York/New Jersey area. The program expanded to Baltimore, and he developed a comparable program in Virginia. Impressed with what Detore had done for high school students, Dr. Filerman brought Mr. Detore to AUPHA to cultivate minority student interest in healthcare management.

From 1970 to 1974, Mr. Detore worked with Haynes Rice and other NAHSE members to provide summer enrichment programs for minority graduate students under the AUPHA umbrella. Dr. Filerman admitted that admission to graduate school was not as significant an issue as graduate placement and practice advancement, over which AUPHA had little influence (Weeks, 1984a).

With three years of funding from the W.K. Kellogg Foundation, AUPHA administered the 11-week summer program (Collins et al., 2008). By the end of the 1973 grant cycle, minority student enrollment in graduate programs was 8.3 percent (Collins et al., 2008). Focusing efforts on increasing the representation of Mexican Americans, Native Americans, and Blacks residing in the South, a new funding initiative was sponsored by the Kellogg Foundation in collaboration with the Robert

Wood Johnson Foundation and the AHA to extend the program through 1975 (G. Filerman, personal communication, January 15, 2018). The grant provided stipends for the student summer work–study program, financial support for AUPHA's Scholarship and Loan Fund for Minority Group Students, and administrative support for AUPHA. Lynette Cooper, AUPHA director of educational opportunities, was responsible for program operations. Additional Kellogg Foundation funding was obtained from 1975 to 1978 (Collins et al., 2008).

In collaboration with NAHSE, AUPHA assumed program management and decided that work–study programs would be based in cities where AUPHA graduate schools were located, thus allowing AUPHA faculty to advise Office of Educational Opportunity staff on how to further develop programs in their respective areas (Weeks, 1984a).

The exception to this site selection was made based on the presence or absence of Mexican and Native American populations and corresponded to underrepresentation of these groups in the local health arena. In spite of aggressive promotion in Los Angeles, San Francisco, San Antonio, and Oklahoma City, programs were not as successful among the Chicano and Native American communities (Weeks, 1984a). A major barrier associated with the Chicano group was believed to be the lack of formal relations with the group prior to initiating the work–study program. Dr. Filerman attributed this in part to the sociology of work–study participants, as well as operational problems within the program (Weeks, 1984a).

AUPHA and NAHSE reported that several cities agreed to participate in the summer program by raising their own funds to pay the student stipends, while others agreed to participate contingent on AUPHA covering program expenses (AUPHA, 1974). Local funding sources, as well as the college work–study program and Urban Corps, were utilized to reduce the expense shared by AUPHA and participating facilities. The Veterans Administration offered full stipend coverage for one student in each of its facilities. In 1976, 17 students were sponsored in Baltimore, Chicago, Newark, New York City, San Francisco, and Seattle (Collins et al., 2008).

AUPHA's goal was to have a decentralized and financially independent network of work–study programs organized at the local level (R. Detore, personal communication, November 15, 2017). At the conclusion of the three-year grant cycle in 1973, only Baltimore, New York, Newark, and San Francisco met the objective of being independent. A total of 241 students participated, with placements in 184 hospitals, neighborhood health centers, family clinics, and health associations (AUPHA, 1974). A survey conducted at the end of the program revealed that 73 percent of students indicated an interest in pursuing a health management career, 48 percent identified health administration as their specific career choice, and the preceptors recommended 86 percent of the participants for the health administration profession (Collins et al., 2008). AUPHA's financial support continued through

1981, and then the local NAHSE chapters assumed responsibility for their respective work–study initiatives.

Over the years, the work–study program grew and contracted. Dr. Filerman reported in his AHA Oral History that at its peak, the summer program operated in 26 cities and provided summer internships for more than 1,400 young people (Weeks, 1984a).

Since hospitals operated as the primary employer for the summer experience, Dr. Filerman and Edwin Crosby, MD, AHA President, negotiated bringing the internship program into AHA before Dr. Crosby's untimely death in 1972. The Institute for Diversity was established in collaboration with ACHE, AHA, and NAHSE. The summer work–study program was subsequently absorbed into AHA. While the increase in minority faculty at the university level was important, the emphasis was on recruiting students and having them recruited by provider organizations.

In 1971, along with helping to establish the summer enrichment program, AUPHA also committed to work with university programs to expand minority graduate enrollment from 3.3 percent to 12 percent over a five-year period (Collins et al., 2008). The Kellogg Foundation, Robert Wood Johnson Foundation, the federal government, Blue Cross Blue Shield, the AHA, the Veterans Administration, and numerous local foundations (Weeks, 1984a) supported outgrowths of the summer program. Coupled with the summer internship, the Robert Wood Johnson Foundation funded graduate education for 100 minority students. The enrollment of minority students in AUPHA programs went from 5 percent in 1977 to 13–15 percent in 1984 (Weeks, 1984a).

REALIZING CHANGE ONE ACTION AT A TIME

There have been several notable efforts to expand diversity in AUPHA's recent past. Following are a few of the highlights.

◆ AUPHA put the issue of diversity on its radar screen in the 1990s after the 1992 landmark joint study by ACHE and NAHSE that compared the career attainments of their members. The report showed that Black healthcare executives with similar education and experience earned lower incomes, held proportionately lower positions, and expressed less job satisfaction than their White counterparts (ACHE, 2008). The study prompted three healthcare organizations, AHA, ACHE, and NAHSE, to create the Institute for Diversity in Health Management. The Association of Hispanic Healthcare Executives joined the Institute shortly after, as did the Catholic Health Association.

- In 1996, Lydia Middleton (Reed) was hired by AUPHA as the director of development. She advanced to become the association's vice president/chief operating officer (COO) and subsequently president/CEO. During Ms. Middleton's 17-year tenure, she focused on financial development, operations, and mission-specific services to the membership, including advancing diversity. From 2001 to 2004, she served as the vice president and COO of the Accrediting Commission on Education for Health Services Administration (ACEHSA) (now known as the Commission on Accreditation of Healthcare Management Education [CAHME]). Ms. Middleton held dual roles at AUPHA and ACEHSA, with the purpose of promoting continuity and economies of scale between the two organizations. In 2004, she was named to *Modern Healthcare*'s 100 Most Influential list. She served on the boards of the Asian Health Care Leaders Association and Institute for Diversity in Health Management, affiliates of AHA.
- Upon her arrival at AUPHA, Ms. Middleton worked to strengthen the faculty forums, particularly the Diversity Forum established in 1999 that has since been renamed the Cultural Perspectives Forum. This group established diversity as an AUPHA Annual Meeting topic.
- Janet Dreachslin, PhD, chaired the AUPHA Diversity Forum from 2000 to 2004 and led the initiative to define domains and core competencies for diversity leadership in health services management. She, along with Augustine Agho, PhD, coauthored the article "Domains and Core Competencies for Effective Evidence-Based Practice in Diversity Leadership" in AUPHA's *Journal of Health Administration Education (JHAE)* (Dreachslin & Agho, 2001).
- In 2001, Raymond Grady presented "The Mandate and Challenge of Increasing Diversity in Healthcare" at the AUPHA Summit on the Future of Education and Practice in Health Management and Policy in Orlando, Florida. He subsequently published the presentation in *JHAE* (Grady, 2001). A key takeaway from the article was that healthcare institutions are an integral part of the social, civic, health, welfare, and economic fabric of society. As such, the leadership of these institutions should reflect the diversity and perspectives of the individuals and families located in the communities they serve. This has been the clarion call for much of the progress made to date in addressing inclusion in the healthcare profession.
- In 2006, Ms. Middleton worked with Hospital Corporation of America (HCA) to introduce the Corris Boyd Scholarship. Mr. Boyd was a senior executive with Health Trust Purchasing Group and HCA who passed away in 2005. The two-year scholarship, established by his widow and HCA,

recognized his leadership and community work by helping finance the education of a student of color who had been accepted to an AUPHA full-member graduate program. At the conclusion of 2017, 25 students from 15 AUPHA-member programs had received this scholarship (AUPHA, 2017b).

- In 2011, diversity was a key addition to the undergraduate program certification standards. Diversity had not been included in previous editions of the program certification standards, so its inclusion was notification to the field that diversity in undergraduate education is important in the recruitment of faculty and students. The criterion is consistent with graduate program accreditation (CAHME, 2017).

- In 2012, Ms. Middleton asked the AUPHA Board for funding for an initiative to develop a diversity and inclusion strategy to improve opportunities for faculty from underrepresented groups in the AUPHA membership (Middleton, 2012). Ms. Middleton worked with the chair of the AUPHA Diversity Faculty Forum, Tondra Moore, PhD, JD, to secure additional funding from the AUPHA Foundation for data collection, analysis, and report preparation. AUPHA funds were matched by the Robert Wood Johnson Foundation. Ms. Middleton's philosophy was that this initiative would drive AUPHA diversity and inclusion efforts and ensure maximum impact, reestablishing a dialog between AUPHA and the foundation on this important issue in the field (Middleton, 2012).

- The results from a comprehensive study of the issues that limit teaching and tenure by underrepresented minorities in healthcare management education (Moore et al., 2013) were presented at the AUPHA Annual Meeting in June 2013. The study analyzed minority faculty teaching in graduate programs and examined minority faculty's workplace perceptions, job satisfaction, mentorship, collaboration, doctoral training, and recommended next steps in advancing the research agenda. The study, commissioned by Ms. Middleton and the AUPHA Board, strengthened the initiatives of the Diversity Faculty Forum.

- In 2012, Ms. Middleton introduced the AUPHA *Body of Knowledge* (AUPHA, 2012) online publication, which delineated the content that students in health management programs should learn during the course of their study. The *Body of Knowledge* was compiled with input from faculty of health management programs throughout the nation. Embedded in the document was a chapter on diversity that listed frequently used texts at the undergraduate and graduate levels.

- The May 30, 2012, AUPHA Board meeting included a discussion of building a diversity agenda. The agenda included diversifying the composition of AUPHA Board members by race, ethnicity, religion, sexual orientation, geography, and employment.

◆ Gerald Glandon, PhD, was selected as AUPHA's President and CEO in 2013 and, through the association's strategic planning mechanism, embedded diversity as a key pillar in the organization's long-term goals (AUPHA, 2016). The diversity initiative was developed into one of the association's five operating committees (see Chapter 11). The committee's goal was to address the ongoing challenge of the lack of diversity among AUPHA member program faculty and students, especially at the graduate level. The committee was charged with developing programs and activities that result in more diversity and inclusion across, among other categories, race, gender, and ethnicity. The thought was that understanding and meeting the challenges of all aspects of diversity would increase membership value and help AUPHA represent the pathway of choice for future leaders. Raymond Grady chaired the committee (AUPHA, 2016).

THE CURRENT PICTURE

In addition to updating the organization's strategic plan, Dr. Glandon led the *Benchmarking and Salary Survey* (AUPHA, 2017a) to gain an appreciation of different member populations. Between 2011 and 2015, the number of program responses to the survey increased from 172 to 220. In 2015, graduate programs reported receiving an average of 94.5 completed applications and made offers to 51.2 of these students on average; 33.5 students matriculated (AUPHA, 2017a). For graduate programs, 64 percent of students are White, 12.8 percent are Black, and 6.6 percent are Hispanic, representing minor decreases in Black and Hispanic student enrollment over the five-year period. Between 2011 and 2015, undergraduate programs saw an increase in full-time students, with one in four students being male. The programs reported that, on average, 53 percent of students are White, 25 percent are Black, and 9 percent are Hispanic (AUPHA, 2017a). (See the following charts.)

The employment picture for graduate and undergraduate students between 2011 and 2015 was sound, with only 6 percent of graduate students and 12 percent of undergraduates still seeking employment or lost to follow-up within three months of graduation (AUPHA, 2017a).

AUPHA reported that between 2011 and 2015, graduate programs had an average of about 15 total faculty, and the median was 14. The largest single category of faculty was adjunct for graduate programs, although this number had decreased over the period. The percentage of female faculty increased from 42.5 percent in 2011

Chart 1. Graduate Student Demographics

	2015 (%)	2011 (%)
Full-time	73.3	66.2
Male	42.9	43.2
White	64.1	61.5
Black	12.8	13.1
Hispanic	6.6	7.3

Chart 2. Undergraduate Student Demographics

	2015 (%)	2011 (%)
Full-time	81.9	65.9
Male	25.3	27.5
White	53.2	51.8
Black	25.1	28.0
Hispanic	8.7	7.5

to 46.7 percent in 2015 (AUPHA, 2017a). The data also suggest that programs are recruiting new individuals to faculty ranks and slowly retiring individuals with substantial years of experience.

The predominant ethnicity of faculty between 2011 and 2015 was White. Most ethnic categories of faculty experienced a slight decline from 2011 to 2015, offset by an increase in the percentage of unreported ethnicity in 2015. It does not appear that AUPHA member programs have been successful in changing the dominant mix of faculty complement during this period (AUPHA, 2017a).

Chart 3. Ethnicity of Program Faculty

Ethnicity	2015 (%)	2011 (%)
White	73.4	77.3
Asian	6.6	9.3
Black	4.1	4.5
Hispanic	1.9	5.3
All other	5.4	3.6

AUPHA moved toward measuring the representation of member programs through its program reviews and surveys. It continues to provide a venue to share diversity and inclusion best practices through its faculty forums. Over the years, AUPHA's focus on diversity and inclusion has evolved. The AUPHA Board has made diversity a strategic imperative, and it promotes diversity in programming through its Cultural Perspectives Faculty Forum, which helps members of the academic community build an inclusive culture. The Forum has become one of AUPHA's most active, with more than 86 members and more than 57 resources posted to the Forum's library.

GUIDELINES FOR IMPROVING DIVERSITY

Healthcare created more jobs than any other sector in 2016, helping to drive total annual job growth to 2.2 million according to data from the U.S. Bureau of Labor statistics. In December 2016 alone, healthcare added 43,200 jobs. The industry accounted for 15.8 million jobs at the end of December 2016 (U.S. Department of Labor, 2017). Healthcare continues to be a leading job producer and a good option for young people seeking careers. However, within those statistics lie continuing opportunities for minorities in clinical and administrative positions. The goal is to create a more balanced workforce that reflects the communities served.

For AUPHA, diversity starts at home. As mentioned earlier, the association included diversity in its 2014 strategic plan as an organizational pillar, along with excellence, innovation, collaboration, and learning. The diversity pillar demonstrates that AUPHA believes in diversity—in people, programs, and perspectives—and feels it is essential for an effective interprofessional workforce. In 2017, the AUPHA Diversity with Inclusion Committee developed the following set of guidelines for building diversity and recommended that academic program directors incorporate these guidelines into their program's strategic plans:

1. Build diversity and inclusion into the strategy of the program with written goals and objectives.
2. Develop an infrastructure to promote diversity, which includes internal and external data that allow the program to measure its performance and compare its progress to others as appropriate.
3. Build diversity into the way programs work every day with policies and procedures. An example might be that for every recruitment effort, a minority candidate should be in the pool of interviewees who are considered for every position.

4. Address the following questions: Does the program have an organizational structure for addressing diversity? An example might be a diversity officer or a link to the university's diversity organizational structure. Does the program foster a culture of diversity in the way decisions are made?

IT TAKES COMMITMENT

AUPHA has a history of leadership in diversity, thanks principally to the leadership of its presidents/CEOs Gary Filerman, PhD, Henry Fernandez, Janet Porter, PhD, Jeptha Dalston, PhD, Lydia Middleton (Reed), MBA, and Gerald Glandon, PhD. Over its 70 years, the association has been involved in strengthening the healthcare management pipeline through internships, scholarships, faculty forums, undergraduate standards, journal publications, its *Body of Knowledge*, and benchmarking surveys. The Board of Directors has also been a driving force, leading the way in promoting diversity in all its forms, including gender, race/ethnicity, sexual orientation, socio-economic status, age, physical abilities, and religious and political beliefs. AUPHA has evolved in its diversity initiatives. It started with student internships in the 1960s and continues to promote student and faculty recruitment with measured success. Looking to the future, we must continue working toward a more diverse faculty and student population, helping expand the pipeline for minority participation in healthcare administration leadership

REFERENCES

American College of Healthcare Executives. (2008). *Coming of age: The 75-year history of the American College of Healthcare Executives*. Chicago, IL: Health Administration Press.

Association of University Programs in Health Administration. (1974). *Work study report*. Washington, DC: Author.

Association of University Programs in Health Administration. (2012). Body of knowledge. Retrieved from http://network.aupha.org/browse/glossary

Association of University Programs in Health Administration. (2016). AUPHA 2016–2019 strategic plan. Retrieved from http://higherlogicdownload.s3. amazonaws.com/AUPHA/5c0a0c07-a7f7-413e-ad73-9b7133ca4c38/Uploaded Images/Strategic_Plan_2016.pdf

Association of University Programs in Health Administration. (2017a). *Benchmarking and salary survey*. Washington, DC: Author.

Association of University Programs in Health Administration. (2017b). Corris Boyd Scholarship. Retrieved from http://network.aupha.org/blogs/chris-sanyer/2017/02/16/corris-boyd-scholarship

Collins, C., Daniels, F., Evans, R., Howard, D., Lofton, M., & Roberts, V. (2008). *The National Association of Health Services Executives: 40 years of breaking the color line in health care management*. Washington, DC: National Association of Health Services Executives.

Commission on Accreditation of Healthcare Management Education. (2017). *Self-study handbook for graduate programs in healthcare management education*. Washington, DC: Author.

Dreachslin, J., & Agho, A. (2001). Domains and core competencies for effective evidence-based practice in diversity leadership. *Journal of Health Administration Education, 19*(Special), 129–145.

Grady, R. (2001). The mandate and challenge of increasing diversity. *Journal of Health Administration Education, 19*(Special), 79–90.

Middleton, L. (2012). *Diversity research proposal. AUPHA Board minutes*. Arlington, VA: Association of University Programs in Health Administration.

Moore, T. L., Elder, K., & Dotson, E. (2013). *Studying issues limiting underrepresented minorities in teaching and tenure in healthcare management*. Arlington, VA: AUPHA/RWJ Foundation.

Sullivan, L. W., & Mittman, S. (2010). The state of diversity in the health professions: A century after Flexner. *Academic Medicine, 85*(2), 246–253.

U.S. Department of Labor. (2017). Databases, tables & calculators by subject. Bureau of Labor Statistics. Retrieved from https://data.bls.gov/pdq/Survey OutputServlet

Weeks, L. (Ed.). (1984a). *Gary Filerman: In first person: An oral history*. Chicago, IL: American Hospital Association.

Weeks, L. (Ed.). (1984b). *Haynes Rice: In first person: An oral history*. Chicago, IL: American Hospital Association.

ABOUT THE AUTHORS

Rupert M. Evans, DHA, FACHE, is Professor and Chairman and Director of the Health Administration Program at Governors State University. He was the President and CEO of the Institute for Diversity in Health Management at the American Hospital Association. Prior to joining the Institute for Diversity, Evans was the President and CEO of the Erie Family Health Center. Erie is one of the largest federally qualified community health centers in Chicago. He is the Chairman of the New Roseland Community Hospital Board of Directors and a member of the Board of Directors of The Leverage Network, Inc., and the Central Michigan University's College of Health Profession Advisory Board. He is a Life Member of Kappa Alpha Psi Fraternity, Inc. Evans is a past president of the Chicago/Midwest Chapter of the National Association of Health Services Executives (NAHSE).

He holds a doctorate of healthcare administration from Central Michigan University, master's degree in public administration/health services management, and bachelor of arts in environmental studies. Dr. Evans is a Fellow of the American College of Healthcare Executives and serves on the AUPHA Board. In March 2017, he was installed as ACHE Regent for the Illinois—Metropolitan Chicago region of ACHE.

Raymond Grady, MHA, FACHE, is the CEO of Methodist Hospitals in Indiana. His prior positions include serving as President of Aurora Healthcare and President of NorthShore University HealthSystem, Evanston Hospital. He served as a member of the Board of Directors for the Indiana Hospital Association and was Chairman of the Board for the American Heart and Stroke Association, Northwest Indiana Chapter. He served on the Board of Directors for AUPHA, AHA Institute for Diversity, Northwest Community Hospital, American Hospital Association, and Illinois Hospital Association. He received his MHA from The Ohio State University and his BS from Morgan State University. Mr. Grady is a Fellow of the American College of Healthcare Executives.

Diane M. Howard, PhD, FACHE, is Associate Professor and Director of Student Development in Health Systems Management at Rush University. Prior to her current role, she was Vice President of Medical Delivery/Director of Contracts at Aetna U.S. Healthcare; Vice President of Medicare, Medicaid, and Individual Products for U.S. Healthcare; Assistant Vice President at Rush Presbyterian St. Luke's Medical Center; and Director of Ambulatory Care for the American Hospital Association. She completed her PhD at the University of Illinois at Chicago, MPH at the University of Pittsburgh, and BA at the Hampton Institute. Dr. Howard is a Fellow of the American College of Healthcare Executives and a former AUPHA Board member.

CHAPTER 6

The Role of Women in AUPHA

Peggy Leatt, PhD,
Janet E. Porter, PhD, and
Mary E. Stefl, PhD

INTRODUCTION

In the early 20th century, women played a major role in hospital management as the number of hospitals grew from 170 in 1870 to about 7,000 by 1925. Hospital beds increased from 35,000 to 860,000 during this same period (Rosner, 1988). Researchers Cynthia Haddock and Nancy Aries noted:

> Early hospital administrators were called "superintendents" and typically had little specific job training—many were nurses who had taken on administrative responsibilities. More than half of the superintendents who belonged to the American Hospital Association in 1916 were graduate nurses. The first formal hospital administration and nursing school administration education program, in health economics, was established for nurses at Columbia Teachers' College in New York in 1900. In addition to the nurses serving in leadership positions, nuns typically ran the burgeoning number of Catholic hospitals. (Haddock & Aries, 1989, p. 33)

Despite this history, hospital administration is one of the few female occupations in the United States that masculinized (Arndt & Bigelow, 2005). Unfortunately, graduate programs in hospital administration actually contributed to this masculinization because they admitted virtually no female students for a long time. As graduate education in hospital administration was established, very few faculty, program directors, or students were female. The early production of only male master of health administration graduates further solidified the image of the hospital administrator as male and the social expectation that a man was required to lead this type of facility (Arndt, 2010).

In this chapter, we describe the incremental involvement of women in the programs designed to educate individuals for hospital administration—and later health administration.

THE DAWN OF A DEGREE: 1920–1940

The first graduate program in hospital administration was started at Marquette University in 1924 and subsequently closed in 1928. The next program launched in 1934 at the University of Chicago. Between 1943 and 1950, 11 programs evolved (seven in schools of public health, two in graduate schools, one in a business school, and one in a college of medicine) (Loebs, 2001). The lack of a specific school location was considered a strength in that it provided opportunities for curricula and faculty diversification. Program development was spurred by young men returning home from war having managed hospitals at the front. They were skilled in hospital operations and saw an opportunity to pass on their knowledge to others.

Passage of the Hill–Burton legislation in 1946 accelerated the construction of hospitals. This led to foundations, policy makers, and academics asking what the requisite skills were for running a hospital. The W.K. Kellogg Foundation played a major role in both answering these questions and providing stimulus funding to establish graduate programs.

THE EMERGENCE OF AUPHA: 1941–1969

It was not until the late 1940s that academic leaders came together to discuss curriculum and admissions standards. On December 17, 1948, the first meeting of the Association of University Programs in Hospital Administration (AUPHA) took place in New York City. Of the 15 persons in attendance, four were women:

- Marguerite Ducker, representing Northwestern University
- Laura G. Jackson, also representing Northwestern University
- Mary Johnson, representing Columbia University
- Eugene Stuart, representing the University of Toronto

The meeting's overall purpose was to establish standard approaches for student admission and curriculum guidelines. Of relevance to women, the minutes indicated "none of the courses (in health administration education programs) bar women but all would be limited to one or two in each class, due mainly to the difficulty in placing women in the field of hospital administration" (AUPHA, 1948, p. 7). This early gender bias would play a significant role in the field's male-dominated evolution.

Between 1949 and 1965, AUPHA was based briefly at Northwestern University and then at the University of Chicago, where faculty developed criteria for admitting programs to the association and created mechanisms for sharing information about member programs. The Kellogg Foundation had played a significant part in establishing the field through study commissions and university grants, and by 1964 it was urging academic leaders to hire full-time leadership for AUPHA. Gary Filerman, PhD, was hired in 1965 as the association's first president and CEO. That year 360 graduate students entered the 28 graduate-level hospital administration programs, but only 34 of these students were women—and many of them came from the church. Half of the 18 programs were all male (Appelbaum, 1975).

Early reflections suggest that hospital administration was basically an occupation for men, where graduates of master's programs claimed the top administration and line management positions, and the fewer women graduates were relegated to staff positions, such as those in planning or research. Some exceptions were in hospitals under church jurisdictions where women's roles were extended from caring to management, especially in Catholic hospitals.

There also was some inherent bias in the way health administration programs were staffed. These kinds of programs were started primarily at universities that were tied to hospitals. When identifying potential faculty and directors for these fledgling health administration programs, the universities typically turned to their respective hospital CEOs and staff, including academics trained in disciplines such as economics, management, or accounting who had an interest in healthcare. There were no doctoral programs in healthcare management to call upon. The vast majority of the faculty were men.

THINGS STARTED TO CHANGE: 1970–1980

By the early 1970s, women started attending hospital administration undergraduate and graduate programs in greater numbers. In 1971, for example, 31 of the 36 graduate programs had female students—although, according to the Accrediting Commission on Education for Health Services Administration (ACEHSA), women represented only 23 percent of graduate students. ACEHSA also reported that in 1973, merely 15 percent of faculty in undergraduate and graduate programs were women.

During this time, AUPHA hired its first female professional staff member. In 1972, Patricia Cahill joined the organization to support AUPHA grants focused on increasing and improving education in mental health administration, long-term care administration, and home health management. During her seven-year tenure, AUPHA grew dramatically, from a staff of 6 to a staff of 19.

In 1973, Marcy Sheinwald did a study of employment patterns of male and female graduate students and found that women were more likely to accept staff positions and positions outside of hospitals than men were. However, women tended to have the same rank, salary, and full-time employment as men. Also in 1973, Edward Spillane studied the disparate careers of men and women in hospital administration in his doctoral dissertation and observed:

> The data reveal that not only is the administrator or top management a "man's world" but the same is true in overwhelming degree of the assistant administrator or upper management levels. Sex is a significant background factor in an individual's chance of achieving an occupational level above a department head in the hospital setting. At the present time, the opportunities for female hospital executives to reach the top of the hospital organizational level are indeed very limited. Present and future hospital executives must be aware of and consider this fact in planning for their hospital administrator careers. (Appelbaum, 1975)

Reflecting the sentiment of the times, Dr. Filerman noted in 1974:

> There is a real difference between the educational opportunities and the employment opportunities (for men and women). The attitudes of hospital management and medical staffs will prevent much of an increase for women in management. It is increasingly less likely a woman will become a CEO of a facility or a program. She must settle in time for less visible roles. (Appelbaum, 1975, p. 58)

Ruth Rothstein, a Chicago hospital executive, attributed this pervasive sentiment to the lack of a visible advocacy group within hospital administration. There was such a group tied to medical practice in the form of the American Medical Women's Association.

As a prelude to what later became known as the *Dixon–Austin Report*, a national conference in 1974 was the culmination of a two-year study that resulted in recommendations to move the two-year graduate curriculum away from a focus on hospitals and toward the broader healthcare system. These changes had the effect of allowing more women to take advantage of job opportunities that emphasized the social/nurturing side of the field (Loebs, 2001).

Although women were underrepresented in hospital leadership positions, there was a significant exception. In 1975, 70 percent of U.S. Catholic hospitals had female administrators, most of whom were members of religious orders, and Catholic hospitals represented 25 percent of the nongovernmental hospitals at that time (Appelbaum, 1975).

The late 1970s brought rapid change in the number of female healthcare management graduates. By 1977–1978, 40 percent of the 1,590 students in the 20 AUPHA undergraduate programs were women, and 39 percent of the 2,917 students in the 65 master's programs were women. Nevertheless, women were significantly underrepresented in academic program leadership, with only two women leading the 20 undergraduate programs (10 percent) and only four women serving as directors of the 65 graduate programs (6 percent) (1979 AUPHA Directory).

THE ROAD TO LEADERSHIP: 1980–1990

During the 1980s, the number of female faculty grew, but female academic leaders were few. From 1987 to 1988, the 30 undergraduate programs were led by seven female directors (23 percent), while 55 percent of the 3,604 students were female. During the same period, only five of the 59 graduate program directors were female (8 percent), while 55 percent of the 5,008 students were women (1989 AUPHA Directory).

Not only were women scarce in program leadership positions, but there also were no women on the AUPHA Board for more than 20 years. However, that changed in 1984 when Peggy Leatt, PhD, became the first female elected to the AUPHA Board. After 39 years of male AUPHA chairs, she became the first female chair from 1987 to 1988. At the same time, Sherril Gelmon, DrPH, was hired as the first female leader of the Accrediting Commission on Education for Health Services Administration (ACEHSA)—the accrediting body (now Commission on Accreditation of Healthcare Management Education [CAHME]) that had been housed within AUPHA since its inception in the 1960s. Dr. Gelmon along with Mary Stefl, PhD, and Kyle Grazier, PhD, had promoted a women's forum in AUPHA to serve as a networking and professional development community for female faculty.

GREATER VISIBILITY FOR WOMEN: 1990–2000

The 1990s saw even more involvement by women in leadership positions in academic programs, as well as AUPHA. Key milestones included the following:

♦ Rosemary Stevens, PhD, of University of Pennsylvania receiving the Baxter Health Services Prize (1990)

- Margaret Mahoney, President of The Commonwealth Fund, delivering the Andrew Pattullo Lecture (1992)
- Carolyn Roberts, CEO of Copley Hospital and first Chair of the American Hospital Association (AHA) Board, being the Abbott Forum Speaker (1996)
- Jacqueline Zinn, PhD, of Temple University being awarded the John D. Thompson Prize for Young Investigators (1996)
- Peggy Leatt, PhD, being named the second recipient of the Gary L. Filerman Prize for Educational Leadership (1997)

During this time, Dr. Filerman was replaced by Henry Fernandez; however, Fernandez resigned in 1998. Janet Porter, PhD, from the University of North Carolina, agreed to serve as Interim CEO for a few months. Realizing that AUPHA had significant financial challenges that had to be resolved before a new CEO could be recruited, Porter led AUPHA for 13 months. Jeptha Dalston, PhD, was then named the third CEO of AUPHA.

During 1997–1998, 22 women led the 35 AUPHA bachelor programs, where 66 percent of the 3,309 students were female. Eighteen women led the 74 graduate programs, where 56 percent of the 5,463 students were female (1999 AUPHA Directory).

The growing role of women in health administration education was explicitly delineated just before the turn of the 21st century. In 1999, AUPHA published a special edition of the *Journal of Health Administration Education* on Women in Health Care Management, edited by Carla Wiggins, PhD. This increased awareness likely led to increased numbers of female students, faculty, and leadership.

Despite the growth of female faculty and administrators in the 1990s, disparities still existed. Steward et al. (1995) found that female administrators had been hired less often than their male peers and had experienced lower levels of job satisfaction, lower status, slower promotion rates, lower salaries, and higher rates of attrition. Stoskope and Xirasagar (1999) surveyed 64 ACEHSA-accredited graduate programs in fall 1997 and found that their ratio of male to female faculty was 1.98, but 2.60 for tenured/tenure-track faculty, despite equal proportions of men and women holding doctorate degrees. Men were more likely to be hired in tenure-track or tenured positions (85 percent), whereas women were hired in tenured positions 71 percent of the time. In addition, men typically were brought on at a higher rank than women, although there was no difference in the extent to which the groups had terminal degrees.

Other interesting facts from the study include the following:

- The schools of public health had more female faculty than the other schools.
- Women were more concentrated in community colleges and less so in more prestigious research-oriented schools.

- Female faculty tended to be more productive (16.9 percent), as measured by a variety of indicators, but received salaries that were 11.3 percent lower than men's. In this study, some women indicated that they were given larger workloads in teaching and administrative work. For example, women tended to assume more counseling and advisory roles than men, which could interfere with more scholarly activities.

Stoskope and Xirasagar (1999) concluded that gender inequality in academia is often rigid, especially around tenure policies, and not designed for flexibility for female roles and lives. They suggested more favorable policies that offer leave, support for child care, and mentoring systems for faculty.

In 1999, Carole Pohl wrote about the glass ceiling as it applies to female faculty in health administration education programs. She noted that women were still underrepresented on health organization boards, in chief executive positions, and at higher ranks in health administration faculty. She found that women outranked men only in the lower levels of the traditional academic hierarchy, such as in the instructor and lecturer levels. Even then, they were likely to be paid at a lower rate than men. Pohl went on to describe how role-modeling and mentoring could help female faculty advancement. Pohl advised young faculty to get involved with activities beyond the traditional academic ones, such as teaching and research, and participate on committees, which can further expand horizons beyond a traditional department or program (Pohl, 1999).

WOMEN'S CURRENT VISIBILITY AND INFLUENCE: 2001– PRESENT

More recently, women have started to play an ever-larger role throughout the field and at AUPHA. For example, in the early 2000s, women began serving as AUPHA committee chairs, forum leaders, Board members, and Board chairs. After Peggy Leatt broke the gender barrier by becoming Board chair, 11 of the next 26 chairs (42 percent) were women (see Table 6.1).

Similarly, more women served as CAHME commissioners, board members, and committee chairs. Peggy Leatt was named chair of the Blue Ribbon Task Force established through funding by the Robert Wood Johnson Foundation. The goal of the group was to evaluate the state of health administration undergraduate and graduate education. This committee's report led to the adoption of competency-based standards. (For more information about this task force and its work, see Chapter 4.)

Table 6.1. Female AUPHA Chairs

Years	Name	Institution
1987–1988	Peggy Leatt, PhD	University of Toronto
1991–1992	Mary E. Stefl, PhD	Trinity University
1992–1993	Deborah Freund, PhD	Indiana University
1995–1996	Cynthia Haddock, PhD	University of Kansas
1996–1997	Mary Richardson, PhD	University of Washington
1998–1999	Janet Reagan, PhD	California State University–Northridge
2004–2005	Diana Hilberman, DrPH	University of California–Los Angeles
2007–2008	Sharon Buchbinder, PhD	Towson University
2012–2013	Sharon Schweikhart, PhD	The Ohio State University
2015–2016	Christy Harris Lemak, PhD	University of Alabama at Birmingham
2016–2017	Diane M. Howard, PhD	Rush University

In 2004, Lydia Middleton (Reed) was named the first female CEO of AUPHA after starting as the association's director of development in 1996. During her nine-year tenure, program membership doubled, and a centralized application process was created for students interested in graduate education programs.

In 2002, AUPHA created the Network Forum on Advancing Women in Healthcare Leadership, which was active in changing the role of women in health administration. By 2017, the network had 122 members, 225 discussion groups, and 37 libraries of materials.

At the same time, women had assumed key leadership roles in the field. During the 2000s, for example, women assumed top spots at *Modern Healthcare*, the American College of Healthcare Executives, and the National Center for Healthcare Leadership.

Also, in 2017, 36 percent of the CAHME-accredited graduate programs and 33 percent of the AUPHA-certified undergraduate programs were led by women. At the same time, half of the AUPHA Board was composed of women.

FACULTY SURVEYS REVEAL GENDER DIFFERENCES

Faculty surveys[1] were conducted intermittently at AUPHA to compare faculty rank, salaries, and benefits. The most recent surveys show some significant changes in the role of women.

In 2001:

- Eighty-six faculty from baccalaureate programs and 183 faculty from graduate programs responded to the survey. Twenty-eight percent were full professors, 22 percent associate professors, 33 percent assistant professors, and 17 percent instructors or lecturers.
- Forty-two percent of the faculty were female and 48 percent male.
- Overall, 44 percent had tenure, and 78 percent were full-time.
- The salaries varied by rank and gender. Full professors, all with tenure, stated salaries were $116,628 per year for men and $80,500 for women (AUPHA, 2001).

By 2007:

- A total of 719 faculty responded to the survey; 32 percent of respondents were professors, 28 percent associate professors, 30 percent assistant professors, and 6 percent instructors/lecturers. Respondents were 40 percent female and 59 percent male.
- Forty-eight percent had 12-month contracts, and 44 percent had 9-month contracts.
- Some faculty were working with graduate programs only (54 percent), some undergraduate only (15.8 percent), and the remainder in both.
- Salaries were almost the same for men and women by 2007. Female professors earned $137,114 annually, and males earned $138,406. Associate professor salaries were the same; males and females earned $102,000. Assistant professors had salaries of $82,000 regardless of gender. Female instructors earned $59,740, whereas male instructors were paid $84,213 (AUPHA, 2007).

By 2012:

- For the 925 respondents to the AUPHA Faculty Survey, the distribution by rank and gender did not change; however, female professors earned $140,346 and males less, $129,029.
- At the associate professor level, females ($91,000) earned slightly more than males ($86,342).
- At the assistant professor level, females and males both earned $81,750. However, at the instructor level, females earned more ($61,801) than males ($58,750) (AUPHA, 2012).

Looking at all three surveys, one sees the growing influence of women in the profession. The 2012 survey results indicate that the stark salary disparity that existed between men and women in 2001 has been vitiated. At this point in our history, women and men are paid substantially the same.

WOMEN'S IMPACT ON THE FIELD

This chapter—and the literature cited within it—points to the fact that the growth of women in academic health administration programs has been relatively slow. However, as the number of programs at both the bachelor and master's level expands, the number of women faculty members has increased.[2]

Unfortunately, this trend has not translated to the field of practice. In its periodic Gender and Careers in Healthcare Management study, the American College of Healthcare Executives (ACHE, 2012) found that women achieved CEO positions at 50 percent of the rate of their male colleagues in 2012. Previous studies (1995 and 2000) showed that women attained CEO positions at 40 percent of the rate for men; the rate was 63 percent in 2006. The 2012 study surveyed healthcare executives with 5–19 years of experience and controlled for time in the field.

Pohl (1999) argues that female faculty members should mentor and provide role models for their junior colleagues. Female faculty may also have a responsibility to provide guidance to their female students as they navigate an environment where the leadership is still dominated by men. The role and impact of women in health administration education and in AUPHA has grown by leaps and bounds. We are reminded by the national culture of our times, however, that more remains to be done with regard to cultivating opportunities and celebrating the achievements both within AUPHA and beyond.

NOTES

1. Because response rates to the surveys were often low, the results are compromised.
2. Unfortunately, the quality and quantity of historical data is limited. For example, for the periods 1943–1950 (first generation), 1950–1966 (second generation), 1966–1973 (third generation), and 1973–2000 (fourth generation), there are few data other than verbal anecdotes. From 2000 to the present, AUPHA directories have not been printed, so data are limited.

REFERENCES

American College of Healthcare Executives. (2012). *A comparison of the career attainments of men and women healthcare executives.* Chicago, IL: Author.

Appelbaum, A. L. (1975). Women in health care administration. Special Report. *Hospitals, 49* (16), 52–59.

Arndt, M. (2010). Education and the masculinization of hospital administration. *Journal of Management History, 16*(1), 75–89.

Arndt, M., & Bigelow, B. (2005). Professionalizing and masculinizing a female occupation: The reconceptualization of hospital administration in the early 1900s. *Administrative Science Quarterly, 50*(2), 233–261.

Association of University Programs in Health Administration. (2001). Faculty salary survey, 2001. Arlington, VA: Author.

Association of University Programs in Health Administration. (2007). Faculty salary survey 2007. Arlington, VA: Author.

Association of University Programs in Health Administration. (2012). Faculty compensation survey 2012. Arlington, VA: Author.

Association of University Programs in Hospital Administration. (1948). Minutes of December 17–19, 1948 meeting. Chicago, IL: Author.

Haddock, C., & Aries, N. (1989). Career development of women in health care administration: A preliminary consideration. *Health Care Management Review, 14*(3), 33–40.

Loebs, S. (2001). The continuing evolution of health management education. *Journal of Health Administration Education Supplement,* Fall, 33–50.

Pohl, C. M. (1999). Promoting career mobility of women faculty in health administration programs. *Journal of Health Administration Education, 17*(2), 83–95.

Rosner, D. (1988). Heterogeneity and uniformity: Historical perspectives on the voluntary hospital. In S. J. Seay & B. C. Vladeck (Eds.), *In sickness and in health: The mission of voluntary health care institutions* (pp. 87–123). New York, NY: McGraw Hill.

Steward, R. I., Patterson, B. T., Morals, P., Bartell, P., Dinas, P., & Powers, R. (1995). Women in higher education and job satisfaction: Does inter-personal style matter? *National Association of Student Personnel Administrators, 33*(1), 43–53.

Stoskope, C. H., & Xirasagar, S. (1999). The glass ceiling in academe: Health administration is no exception. *Journal of Health Administration Education, 17*(2), 67–82.

ABOUT THE AUTHORS

Peggy Leatt, PhD, was Professor and Chair of the Department of Health Policy and Management at the University of Toronto for 10 years (1981–1991). In this position she was also CEO of the Health Services Restructuring Commission of Ontario, advising the minister of health on health policy. From 2001 to 2013, she was Professor and Chair of the Department of Health Policy and Management at the University of North Carolina at Chapel Hill.

Janet E. Porter, PhD, served as Interim President of AUPHA from 1997 to 1998. She has been active in Commission on Accreditation for Healthcare Management Education for 20 years, serving as a Fellow, Commissioner, Board Member, and Chair of the Standards Council. She is currently an Adjunct Professor at the University of Miami, University of North Carolina, and The Ohio State University, where she is also a member of the Board of Trustees. Janet is the former Chief Operating Officer of Nationwide Children's Hospital and Dana-Farber Cancer Institute and the former Associate Dean of Gillings School of Public Health at the University of North Carolina at Chapel Hill.

Mary E. Stefl, PhD, was Professor and Chair of Trinity University's Department of Health Care Administration from 1987 to 1994 and 2001 to 2013. She is a past chair of AUPHA and has a long history with accreditation, having chaired the Board of Directors of the Commission on Accreditation for Healthcare Management Education as well as its predecessor organization, the Accrediting Commission on Education for Health Services Administration.

CHAPTER 7

Expanding Health Administration Globally: The Role of AUPHA

Bernardo Ramirez, MD,
William E. Aaronson, PhD, and
Daniel J. West Jr., PhD, FACHE

INTRODUCTION

The Association of University Programs in Health Administration (AUPHA) was organized primarily to support the development of healthcare (originally "hospital") management education in the United States and Canada. However, early in its development, the association took advantage of existing international relationships, growing health systems development support, and interest in comparative systems to support its primary mission of strengthening healthcare administration education internationally. International program development was largely supported by foundations, the U.S. federal government, and international health agencies as the role of health administration education coincided with their agendas.

This chapter provides an overview of the evolution of international health management education initiatives, programs, and activities facilitated by AUPHA, member programs, and faculty. The intent is to describe the role that international engagement has played in advancing the AUPHA mission. The chapter will also show the impact global engagement has had on the member programs and their faculties.

The diversification of the population, the multinational character of many healthcare businesses, and the importance of health in international development compel faculty and students of healthcare management to understand how societies organize to meet the health needs of their populations and their approaches to management.

To some, AUPHA's involvement in international activities has been viewed as a distraction from the organization's main purpose. Those who have been involved with AUPHA-sponsored and facilitated international activities believe the impact of this involvement has made a substantial contribution to the professional development of our faculty and of our programs. It has not been a distraction but has come to be a significant element in the association's development.

THE EARLY YEARS

The W.K. Kellogg Foundation was the key source of support for the development of the health administration profession not only in the United States and Canada, but also in Latin America, Australia, and Europe. Mr. Andrew (Andy) Pattullo from the Kellogg Foundation informally participated on the AUPHA Executive Committee since the early years of the association, providing support and resources for many AUPHA International initiatives. Initial interest in programs outside the United States and Canada manifested in 1964, when AUPHA received a five-year grant from the Kellogg Foundation to expand the international activities of the association. The grant included support for an executive director and the development of curriculum committees. AUPHA's leadership visited a new program at the University of Mexico and subsequently began a discussion about establishing an associate membership category for programs in Latin America. A representative of the Mexican program, Dr. Antonio Vila, and a guest from the University of Venezuela, Dr. Pedro Garcia Clara, were invited to attend the AUPHA meeting in August of that year (AUPHA, 1964).

Gary Filerman, because of his keen interest in and knowledge of the Latin American healthcare systems and of healthcare management education and practice, pursued an international vision for AUPHA. In the late 1960s and early 1970s, Gary Filerman had a master's degree in Latin American Government and, as a Kellogg and Organization of American States fellow, had written his doctoral thesis in Chile, conducting a study of the organization of the Chilean National Health Service, mentored by Dr. Fidel Urrutia and Rafael Plisscoff. AUPHA grew its number of members, thereby stimulating the creation of new task forces, collaboration opportunities, and other initiatives. Because the AUPHA mission and capacity aligned with the Kellogg Foundation's objectives, there was a natural convergence of interests. (AUPHA, 1965b).

FIRST INTERNATIONAL ACTIVITIES: EMPHASIS ON LATIN AMERICA

In the 1940s the economic development of the hemisphere became an important American policy objective. By the 1950s there was growing recognition of the importance of Latin American healthcare systems in development and the need to provide sustained and multifaceted support that went beyond the traditional emphasis on the public health infrastructure. Much of the early development work in both public health and health systems was based in the Pan American Health Organization (PAHO), with Kellogg Foundation support. PAHO started in 1902, before the WHO in 1945, and serves as the specialized health agency for the inter-American system and also as the regional office for the Americas of the WHO, the specialized health agency of the United Nations (PAHO, n.d.).

The Kellogg Foundation began supporting health (hospital) administration programs in 1950 with the graduate program at the University of Sao Paulo. During the 1950s and 1960s, Latin American countries developed a substantial number of hospitals with state-of-the-art technology necessitating well-trained health administrators. By the mid-1960s there were university programs in Argentina, Brazil, Chile, Colombia, Mexico, Peru, Puerto Rico, and Venezuela. All but Puerto Rico had benefited from Kellogg support, mainly in the form of faculty fellowships at U.S. and Canadian universities. Most of these programs were in schools of public health or medicine. Others were located in ministries of health, social security organizations, or hospital associations and offered short-term courses with part-time faculty. The university-based programs developed close relations with AUPHA and with several member programs through the faculty exchanges, participation in AUPHA meetings, and related organizations such as the American Hospital Association, the American College of Hospital Administrators, and PAHO (DeVries, Kisil, & Ramirez, 1988).

With Kellogg Foundation encouragement in the mid-1960s, AUPHA developed a close collaboration with PAHO, which continued for 20 years. By 1965 the Kellogg Foundation was supporting several programs in Latin America, most notably those based at the University of Sao Paulo in Brazil, founded and headed by Dr. Odair Pedroso; the University of Venezuela, headed by Dr. Pedro Garcia Clara; and the National Autonomous University of Mexico, headed by Dr. Antonio Rios Vargas. The association's initiatives began with representatives of these programs participating in AUPHA meetings and activities (AUPHA, 1965a).

In August 1966, in collaboration with the Pan-American Federation of Associations of Medical Schools (PAFAMS) and with Kellogg Foundation support, AUPHA convened the first Latin American Conference in Hospital Administration Education in Bogota, Colombia. Seventeen faculty and program directors from 9 countries (Argentina, Brazil, Canada, Chile, Colombia, Mexico, Peru, the United States, and Venezuela) and Puerto Rico attended. The following members represented AUPHA at this meeting: Dr. F. Burns Roth, University of Toronto; John Thompson, Yale University; Lawrence Hill, University of Michigan; Dr. Guillermo Fajardo, University of Mexico; and Gary Filerman, president and CEO, AUPHA (AUPHA, 1967). Attendees sought to improve the relationships among the programs and develop a system for the exchange of state-of-the-art teaching techniques and curriculum materials. In addition, they sought to discern "patterns of education in hospital administration throughout the world." Since most countries had only one program, isolation and faculty inbreeding were serious problems. Conference presentations included mapping health administration education programs and surveys of practice issues, resources, and perspectives. Improved relationships and communication among the participants was the main achievement of the conference. Given the increasing interest of international activities, an AUPHA Committee on International Activities started working at the 1967 Annual Meeting. The members of the committee were F. Burns Roth, University of Toronto; Ralph Murray, St. Louis University; Allan Caldwell, University of California–Los Angeles; and Leon Gintzig, The George Washington University (AUPHA, 1966c).

In 1967, AUPHA leadership and faculty participated in several exploratory visits and a regional meeting in collaboration with PAHO. Two regional meetings advanced these collaborations. In February a Board meeting continued to consider the possible membership of the program in Mexico City, and in August PAHO sponsored a Latin American Conference on Teaching Medical Care Administration at the National School of Public Health in Medellin, Colombia (AUPHA, 1967).

In 1975, in part stimulated by the report of the Commission on Education for Health Administration (Dixon Report) and the Kellogg Foundation, PAHO undertook an assessment of Latin American health administration education that included a review of the status of the 44 programs identified in the region. This study resulted in Kellogg supporting a second generation of investments under the PROASA (Advanced Programs in Health Administration Education) program, which was coordinated by PAHO. The Kellogg Foundation investment was $5.5 million over 10 years. Selected programs developed 10 projects, each of which designated a center of excellence for a specific topic or approach to health management education. Centers were to develop that capacity in the other programs through workshops, conferences, development of materials, and exchange of faculty and students (DeVries et al., 1988).

The common characteristics of these centers of excellence were as follows:

1. Innovation in the teaching of health administration as evidenced in the kind of training offered, curricular design, teaching methods, incorporation of new disciplines, and the development of teaching materials;
2. Use of systemic studies to determine managerial needs, impact of prepared managers in health services delivery, and the development of alternative innovative models for the provision of health services;

3. Use of consortium-type interaction between diverse academic settings (health administration) and health service organizations. (DeVries et al., 1988, p. 924)

Between 1976 and 1987, 10 programs developed across Latin America with the following emphases:

- In Brazil, two programs were initiated: one at The Getulio Vargas Foundation in Rio de Janeiro with emphasis in Public Administration and Policy; and a consortium between the Getulio Vargas Foundation School of Business in Sao Paulo and the Hospital das Clinicas of the University of Sao Paulo, with an emphasis on administrative residencies and a strong innovative business curriculum.
- Two programs began operating in Colombia: one at Universidad del Valle in Cali with emphasis in social medicine with an interdisciplinary approach and strong links to the regional and state health services; the second one in the Javeriana University in Bogota, located in an interdisciplinary college with strong emphasis on social security administration.
- In Chile, at the University of Chile in Santiago, the program was established as a consortium between the business school and the school of public health that created a combined program modernizing the curriculum of the school of public health.
- In Argentina, the program at the University of Buenos Aires School of Architecture and Urban Planning had an architectural/managerial approach to healthcare facilities.
- In the Dominican Republic, the program in Santiago de los Caballeros at the Catholic University Madre y Maestra explored undergraduate education modalities to improve the public hospitals.
- In Mexico, the program contributed to the modernization of the School of Public Health and brought health services research to support the development of the National Institute of Public Health.
- In Peru, the program developed in the Cayetano Heredia Peruvian University helped modernize medical healthcare and public health management.
- The 10th program was in San Jose, Costa Rica, at the Central American Institute of Public Administration. It served students from the Central American region, providing education in public policy with strong managerial content in the health sector organizations.

The PROASA program was continually evaluated. A mid-term evaluation in March 1980 showed the program had provided support for educators and students in 58 advanced health administration courses from 35 institutions in 14 countries. The evaluation also proposed permanent literature reference systems and the dissemination of more teaching materials and health services research. The AUPHA executive director was a member of the advisory committee and developed a number of collaborations, including presentations at annual meetings (PAHO, 1983).

An office of International Health Administration Education was established in 1980 to address the areas highlighted in the PAHO evaluation and to strengthen AUPHA's international activities. This office was led by Robert (Bob) Emrey, who after his tenure in AUPHA became an officer of the Agency for International Development and continued to support health administration education.AUPHA had been actively promoting international program membership, and by then had 66 international members, including 23 Latin American programs. Some of the key initiatives included the strengthening and expansion of the AUPHA Resource Center, expanding the international scope of the *Journal of Health Administration Education*, and incorporating Latin American and international faculty members in curriculum development task forces and other AUPHA activities (AUPHA, 1981).

AUPHA AND THE WORLDWIDE DEVELOPMENT OF HEALTH ADMINISTRATION EDUCATION

The post–World War II era brought the establishment of the National Health Service (NHS) in the United Kingdom, development of payment systems and social health insurance in Europe, and later the establishment of the Medicare and Medicaid programs in the United States. These advances created the need for professional management in healthcare organizations. Bureaucratization and corporatization of healthcare delivery demanded a new class of managers. The establishment of the second and third waves of health administration programs in the United States and Canada is discussed elsewhere in this book.

In the late 1950s and early 1960s, interest in health/hospital management education grew rapidly in Europe and Australia. Because the United States and Canada were recognized for the quality of their management education, it was natural to seek the assistance of AUPHA member programs in establishing health administration programs. In Britain, the King's Fund was the primary resource for management development for the NHS, offering a range of short courses for administrators of various services. The Fund also hosted the annual Hospital Conference of Western Europe, an important vehicle for continuing education and networking. The NHS, with the support of the Fund, developed a plan for a national university-based training scheme. That plan led to the development of programs in five universities, with particularly influential programs at the universities of Manchester, Birmingham, and Leeds. The AUPHA executive Dr. Gary Filerman was a consultant to the NHS planning committee and participated in some of the conferences.

Several programs developed in Europe in the 1960s. The University of Leuven, Belgium, created an influential program/research center with the mission of supporting the development of educational programs and health policy throughout the European Union. The center had a close tie to AUPHA, with Dr. Filerman serving as a consultant for two months. Programs also were developed at the French and Portuguese national schools of public health, the Norwegian School of Local Government and Social Work, and the Nordic School of Public Health, among others. Unlike the Latin American experience, the European program leaders were well known to each other and had significant interactions.

In 1979, the Kellogg Foundation provided initial support for the European Association of Programmes in Health Services Studies (EAPHSS) that was established in Dublin, Ireland (DeVries et al., 1988). The association was modeled after AUPHA, and the grant included support for AUPHA's executive, Dr. Gary Filerman, to spend time at the association office, visit programs, and attend annual meetings. Initially composed of health administration academic programs, the EAPHSS evolved to include in its membership a variety of healthcare organizations and a focus on health policy and health professions education. By the time of the publication of its 1990 *Directory of Membership*, the organization had changed its name to the European Health Management Association (EHMA, 1990). EHMA is located in Brussels, Belgium, consistent with its close interactions with other European Union organizations.

The Institute of Hospital Administrators, now the Australian College of Health Service Executives (ACHSE), started a diploma program in health administration in 1945 and continues to play a key partnership role with the Society for Health Administration Programs in Education (SHAPE). In 1956, with the support of the Kellogg Foundation, the University of New South Wales in Sydney established a new school of hospital administration that developed the country's first university master's degree program in health administration (Grant, 1991). In the early 1980s, the Kellogg Foundation supported visits to Australia by its program director, Andrew Pattullo, and two AUPHA program directors. As a result, the foundation provided support for the establishment of SHAPE, based at the South Australian Institute of Technology in Adelaide, in 1985. AUPHA served as the model. SHAPE included programs at the University of New South Wales, the University of Sydney, Curtin University in Perth, the Western Australian Institute of Technology, Queensland Institute of Technology, Royal Melbourne Institute of Technology, and Massey

University in New Zealand (SHAPE, 2017). These are the initial programs that were members of SHAPE. The history of SHAPE can be found at http://www.shape.org.au/wp-content/uploads/2011/05/SHAPE-History1.pdf, and a current list of member programs at http://www.shape.org.au/program-directory/.

While Latin America, Europe, and Australasia were AUPHA's primary international foci during the 15 years from 1965 to 1980, it facilitated engagement with emerging programs in Africa, Asia, and the Middle East.

AUPHA SPONSORS INTERNATIONAL FACULTY DEVELOPMENT INSTITUTES

AUPHA's 1966 Annual Meeting included a discussion of creating international faculty institutes (AUPHA, 1966b). Previously, the association had established "curriculum committees" to share and develop basic components of the program curriculum (AUPHA, 1964). In March 1966 the AUPHA Executive Committee considered the development of faculty institutes on Teaching Medical Care (one of the three initial curriculum committees), the Role of the Hospital in Medical Care, and Hospital Organization and Hospital Planning. These institutes were considered to prepare AUPHA for participation in an Institute on Medical Care to be convened by the health field as a whole. The Institute on Medical Care would focus on the changing pattern of institutional and extra-institutional relationships in the delivery of medical care (AUPHA, 1966a).

In 1967, Gary Filerman, while raising funds for the expanding AUPHA activities, received a gift from Foster McGaw, the founder of the American Hospital Supply Corporation, to support an international faculty development fund. The fund provided travel fellowships for faculty members from international affiliates to visit U.S. and Canadian programs to discuss faculty development and curricular issues, culminating with participation at the AUPHA Annual Meeting. Two faculty members participated annually until the 1980s (Weeks, 1983).

Starting in 1971, AUPHA expanded the faculty institutes. The objective was to strengthen teaching and research in comparative health systems by exploring in depth a foreign health system. U.S. and Canadian faculty visited programs for an intensive two- to three-week period to exchange ideas and create research and teaching interest bonds with their counterparts (Weeks, 1983). The first AUPHA international faculty institute took place in London in 1971 and was hosted by the King's Fund College. It provided an opportunity for AUPHA members to interact with University of Leuven faculty and later to contribute to the development of the Institute for European Health Services Research in Belgium in 1972 (AUPHA, 1972).

The second AUPHA international faculty institute was cosponsored with PAHO and supported by a Kellogg Foundation grant. It took place at Carleton University in Ottawa, Canada, in 1973. Fifty faculty members from the United States and several Latin American programs participated. The third such institute focused on the organization of health services in Finland. Held in Helsinki, Finland, in 1973, it was hosted by the Finland Hospital Association and the Ministry of Health. Faculty from the United States and other countries participated in a multinational comparison of decision-making decentralization, rational allocation of resources, and cost containment ideas. Several of the participants also traveled to Copenhagen for a three-day orientation to the role of the World Health Organization (WHO) in Europe and to participate in a regional workshop titled "Evaluation of Screening Programs/Epidemiology and Primary Care/Use of Hospital Data" (AUPHA, 1975).

One important result of these AUPHA international faculty institutes was the growing interest in comparative healthcare systems. The interest also stimulated the publication of an initial textbook in this area by the Health Administration Press (Roemer, 1976). The press was established in 1972 with the support of the W.K. Kellogg Foundation as a joint endeavor of AUPHA (Washington, DC) and the Cooperative Information Center for Hospital Management Studies (University of Michigan). This first textbook was a collection of 30 papers developed by Milton Irwin Roemer during his 25 years of field experiences. The book's foreword was written by Dr. Karl Evang, Director General of Health Services of Norway. He remarked that prior to this publication, only a very limited number of readers had access to such materials. With this publication, a larger audience of scholars had access to this growing area.

One of the seminal international activities that propelled and further strengthened AUPHA's global network of faculty and programs was the fourth AUPHA international faculty institute and the First International Course on Education for Health Services Administration held in Portugal in 1981. The course was cosponsored by AUPHA, EAPHSS, and the National School of Public Health of Portugal (NSPH) with support from WHO, the Portuguese Ministry of Social Affairs, and the Calouste Guilbenkian Foundation. Twelve other organizations and foundations, including the Kellogg Foundation, contributed support, including scholarships. Eighty-seven leaders and educators from 29 countries participated in a three-day institute with WHO and national experts to explore issues and trends of health systems worldwide. Eight days of conferences, workshops, and other interactive activities focused on key problems and opportunities facing healthcare management faculty and programs in Africa, Europe, Asia, North and South America, and Australia. Key areas of study were assessing the national need for health administration; case studies of education for health administrators in Europe, Latin America, the Philippines, the socialist countries, and the United States; curriculum content development; and organizing clinical experience and nontraditional programs (AUPHA, 1981; NSPH, 1983). A substantial publication containing the presentations from the international faculty institute was distributed worldwide by AUPHA. During the second week of the institute, participants divided into small groups that visited eight regions of Portugal to observe their healthcare system and management practices.

USAID COOPERATIVE AGREEMENTS

Starting in the early 1990s, AUPHA pursued a number of initiatives with the U.S. Agency for International Development (USAID) to develop and implement healthcare management education in various regions. These cooperative agreements were all unique but helped AUPHA pursue its goal of expanding health administration education globally.

The Latin American Development Program: 1985–1994

In 1985, AUPHA entered into a cooperative agreement with USAID to develop a program aimed at strengthening health administration education in Latin America and the Caribbean (LAC). Bernardo Ramirez, MD, directed this program and the AUPHA Office of International Development from 1985 (AUPHA, 1986) and also served as Vice President from 1992 to 1999 (AUPHA, 1992).The program had the following objectives:

1. To serve as facilitator for USAID mission and host country consumers of health management training and technical assistance and to support training centers and technical assistance providers
2. To provide communication channels between and among U.S. and Latin American health management training centers
3. To assist Latin American health management training centers to improve the relevance, applicability, and responsiveness of training needs for health management (AUPHA, 1985)

The program was initially approved for four years and after a successful midterm evaluation was extended for one more year (AUPHA, 1989). At the end of this initial period, the cooperative agreement was extended for another five years. Activities included the following:

1. The collection, publication, and dissemination of health management training resources and other relevant materials to USAID missions, host country health organizations, and health management training institutions
2. The development and maintenance of a directory of U.S. and LAC health management training institutions and an index of specialists with health management skills
3. The delivery of a maximum of two months of consultant site visits per year to train or assist in identifying management training needs, including assisting in matching those training needs with appropriate partner programs
4. Enlarging and maintaining the network of healthcare management education institutions in the region

In other words, the agreement provided support for the full range of AUPHA program development objectives in the region.

AUPHA operated field offices in San Jose, Costa Rica, from 1989 to 1991 (AUPHA, 1989) and in Bogota, Colombia, in partnership with the Colombian Association of Universities from 1992 to 1998. Annually, the LAC program implemented at least one regional workshop and a combination of several subregional or national topic-specific workshops. The publication and dissemination program included semiannual newsletters; the expansion and maintenance of a resource center with a reference collection of teaching materials and bibliographies on health administration education; and translation, publication, and distribution of the *Journal of Health Administration Education* (*JHAE*) and quarterly special reports. A Spanish-language supplement was included in *JHAE* beginning with issue 4, number 1, in 1986 to issue 13, number 2, in 1995.

When the USAID support for the LAC program ended in 1997, AUPHA continued its commitment to the region, supporting basic activities by using the Internet, electronic publications, and the partnerships developed through the years. When funding was discontinued, there were programs in virtually all of the region's countries. Many Canadian and U.S. faculty members had participated, and direct program-to-program collaborations had been established (AUPHA, 1998).

USAID Cooperative Agreements and Grants in the Newly Independent States and Central and Eastern Europe: 1994–2000

In 1988, the Solidarity Movement won a free election in Poland that marked the beginning of the end of communist rule in Central and Eastern Europe (CEE) and the Soviet Union. That alone should not have had an impact on U.S. healthcare or health administration education. However, one of the pillars of Leninism was universal access to healthcare. With the imploding economies of the Soviet Union and CEE, a major concern arose among European nations and the United States. The Semashko centralized healthcare system, named after Dr. Nikolai Semashko, Minister of Health of the Soviet Union (1918–1930), brought advances in population health that lasted until the 1970s, when it started emphasizing specialization in hospital and outpatient care. The USSR was "one of the first countries to achieve something close to universal coverage of basic health-care services" (Sheiman, 2013). The fear was that the Semashko system of public health and healthcare delivery would collapse and exacerbate the potential for civil unrest and chaos.

The United States made a major commitment to support the transition of the formerly communist nations to market economies and to prop up the imploding healthcare delivery systems. USAID was given the major responsibility to identify and meet the needs for transition planning. To complicate matters, the healthcare systems in the Soviet Union and in much of CEE had been neglected for decades. Any attempt to improve healthcare institutions delivering care would require transformation of management practice.

AUPHA and the AIHA Health Partnership Programs

The American International Health Alliance (AIHA) was formed through the initiative of USAID to support a novel partnership concept based on a consortium of major healthcare provider organizations, including AUPHA (AIHA, 2017). AIHA is an independent nonprofit corporation. In 1992, AIHA and USAID agreed to support a partnership program pairing hospitals in the United States with hospitals in the New Independent States (NIS) of the former Soviet Union. Dr. Lee Hougan was an alumnus of the doctoral program and faculty member in Public Health at Tulane University. He had supported AUPHA International activities as a Project Officer of USAID since the 1980s on Latin America initiatives, where he was the USAID representative for the Dominican Republic. He was the agency's leader in the development of the AIHA partnership program and in integrating health administration into the core activities of all the projects. He retired in 1994 as described in the article "I wanted to get involved," published by AIHA in the *CommonHealth* (AIHA, 1994). The health partnership programs were fashioned after the Marshall Plan to provide training and support to rebuild health services and social systems in the NIS and in CEE, which had been dominated by the Soviet Union in the post-war era.

The AIHA partnership model included the following features:

♦ A partnership connecting one or more U.S. and NIS/CEE institutions with common interests and purposes
♦ Volunteers providing technical assistance and training to partners
♦ Exchange visits in both directions
♦ Giving partners broad exposure to healthcare systems
♦ Peer-to-peer relationships at the institutional level
♦ Financial and technological resources donated by U.S. partners to NIS/CEE partners
♦ AIHA managing the logistics of the partnerships

The partnerships were to assist in modernizing technology and updating clinical care with a focus on nursing, infection control, women's health, neonatal resuscitation, and emergency medicine. Patient-centered care was introduced to hospitals, and nongovernmental organizations were founded to address social, psychological, and economic concerns.

The partnership concept was later expanded to include other types of healthcare organizations, health insurance programs, ministries of health, and healthcare management educational institutions.

Health Management Training in Support of AIHA Partnerships

In 1993, AIHA and AUPHA reached an agreement to provide much-needed management training to the partners in the NIS/CEE region. The purpose was to provide hospital leadership with the competencies and tools to transform their organizations and benefit from the AIHA-sponsored partnerships. AUPHA first developed a series of management training curriculum modules that became known as Management 101: Introduction to Management. These courses were supplemented with a book developed by several AUPHA faculty members. This book was an effort by AUPHA to provide all the important topics of applied health administration to promote the field in the United States and internationally. The editors were Robert Taylor and Susan Taylor. A large number of AUPHA faculty were contributors and advisers (Taylor & Taylor, 1994). The management training manual became very popular with AUPHA's international partners, since it was a comprehensive review of applied healthcare management (Breindel, 1994). The process of module development involved numerous AUPHA faculty members. The modules had an executive education format designed to engage participants in applying new knowledge and skills immediately. While familiar to AUPHA faculty, this approach to education was new for the participants in the NIS/CEE region. The modules were translated into Russian and multiple CEE languages (Ramirez, Perfiljeva, & Voronenko, 1994).

AUPHA then recruited faculty to teach one- to two-week workshops in the NIS/CEE region. This required expansion of the AUPHA international office and the development of mechanisms to invite, screen, and train faculty from AUPHA member programs who then served as faculty in the workshops. This effort was led by Bernardo Ramirez, AUPHA Vice President, and William Aaronson, of Temple University. The training focused not only on the content, but also on teaching cross-culturally and becoming proficient in working with translators. Thus, faculty who participated increased their international and cultural competence at a time when those skills were of growing importance in the United States (Ramirez & Schreiber, 1995).

In recognition of the limitations of such an approach, AUPHA developed a "train the trainers" program for participants in the NIS/CEE to propagate the training program through deployment of local faculty in each of the countries. In addition, AUPHA member faculty developed financial and quality management workshops to provide opportunities for participants to further advance their skills.

An assessment of these programs showed that the collaborative and participatory approach of the AIHA model brought sustainable results at the personal, professional, institutional, and policy levels in the NIS/ CEE countries. Many of these partnership sites provided important cultural changes through the use of volunteerism, modern communication technology, partnership approaches, and a "bottom-up" collaborative approach (USAID, 2006; AIHA, 2017).

From the beginning, women, mostly physicians and nurses, were very active in the partnerships and were part of the management teams that participated in the management training workshops and activities. Many of them noted that the clinical ideas exchange had been useful, but the most significant achievement was their role as more active members of the healthcare management teams. To disseminate the women's elevated role in management, AUPHA/AIHA produced a video entitled "Women Leaders: Changing Healthcare in the NIS," which was distributed during the annual meeting of the partnerships in Iowa. Eight distinguished alumni from the management training courses who had led management teams in several of the participating countries developed this project with Dr. Elena Bourganskaia and Susan Taylor (AIHA, 1996)

DEVELOPING HEALTHCARE MANAGEMENT EDUCATIONAL PROGRAMS THROUGH UNIVERSITY PARTNERSHIPS

Academic partnerships have long linked American scholars with scholars in other countries. The Fulbright Program was established in 1946 (U.S. Department of

State, 2017). The International Research and Exchanges Board (IREX, 2017) was founded in 1968 to facilitate the development of and access to education worldwide through scholar and student exchanges. IREX and AUPHA later joined forces in supporting a new exchange concept.

The AUPHA-IREX Partnership program in Russia was initiated in 1994. The project paired three AUPHA member universities with universities in the Russian Federation. AUPHA was the principal organization in partnership with IREX. However, AUPHA entered into a subagreement with AIHA to provide the logistical arrangements for these partnerships and in-country activities supported by the AIHA Russian office and staff. The program's objective was to strengthen indigenous capacity in health administration education in Russia to support health reform and improve the quality and performance of healthcare organizations. Three partnerships were established, between (1) the Moscow Medical Stomatology Institute and Tulane University, (2) the Novosibirsk State Academy for Economics and Management and the University of Washington, and (3) the Far East Medical Academy in Khabarovsk and the University of Kentucky. This AUPHA program of partnerships was designed and developed with a national Association of Educational Programs in Health Administration hosted by the Sechenov Medical Academy in Moscow (Counte, Aaronson, & Ramirez, 2001).

AIHA further recognized that healthcare management education would need to be developed in the other target countries to advance the development of professional managers. In 1995, USAID asked AIHA to expand the partnership twinning concept by soliciting American healthcare management programs to partner with universities in CEE that expressed an interest in developing healthcare management programs. The Health Management Education (HME) partnership has had a lasting effect on the AUPHA member programs involved. With AUPHA's assistance, five member programs were identified through an open solicitation. The U.S. programs were paired with universities in the Czech Republic, Slovakia, Romania, and Albania. AUPHA provided professional support to the new partnerships.

For the results of the HME partnership project to be disseminated, the USAID/AIHA cooperative agreement provided funding to AUPHA to publish two special issues of the *Journal of Health Administration Education*. The two special issues, published in 1997 and 1998, respectively, focused on the introduction of health management education in the CEE region and emphasized the role that AUPHA and member programs played in the process (Aaronson, & West, 1997, 1998).

The Slovakia HME partnership produced numerous programs in health management education at the undergraduate and post-graduate levels. The University of Scranton (UoS) continues the partnership with St. Elizabeth University and Trnava University in Slovakia. The UoS developed what is known as "The Bridge

Model" and implemented similar sustainable projects using the university-based partnership model in Africa; Mexico; and Tbilisi, Georgia.

THE IMPACT OF THE AUPHA/AIHA PARTNERSHIP

The evaluation of the impact of the USAID/AIHA health partnership programs noted that the health partnerships approach "fostered a sense of equality among partners." The overall development impact of the AIHA partnerships involving AUPHA member universities demonstrated that the partnership approach can be used as a tool of foreign assistance and that institutional change can be achieved as an objective of the partnership model. An additional finding was that changes in healthcare and social systems could be achieved at a systemwide level using HME partnerships (USAID, 2006; Counte, Ramirez, & Aaronson, 2011; Aaronson, West, Heshmat, & Ramirez, 1998; Aaronson, 1997; Aaronson, Counte, & Ramirez, 2008).

While the results of the AIHA partnerships supported by AUPHA had demonstrable benefits to the nations emerging from decades of underfunding and misguided management, there were also numerous benefits that accrued to AUPHA member programs. The management training project involved roughly 50 faculty members from 10 AUPHA member programs. Many faculty members experienced a cultural awakening and a better understanding of what it means to be globally competent.

Participation in the USAID-sponsored project was made possible when AUPHA joined the USAID/AIHA partnership project in the NIS and CEE regions. This project had a profound influence on AUPHA and on AUPHA member programs and faculty, largely because of the large number of faculty who engaged in the project. Although these projects were completed by 2000, the interest in global health management continued to grow among programs and faculty. In the absence of external funding, faculty instead advanced global health management education largely through more traditional means and voluntary efforts to sustain this focus within AUPHA. By the end of the project, there were programs in virtually all of the region's countries. Many Canadian and U.S. faculty members had participated, and direct program-to-program collaborations had been established.

AUPHA GLOBAL HEALTH MANAGEMENT EDUCATION DEVELOPMENT INITIATIVES: 2000–2017

After 2000, AUPHA continued to pursue health management initiatives through a series of partnerships and internal initiatives. These built upon the earlier efforts done collaboratively with USAID and represent a model for the future.

European Academy of Management

The Global Healthcare Management Faculty Forum (GHMFF) initiated a plan to participate in the European Academy of Management (EURAM). EURAM is a community of engaged scholars dedicated to developing responsible research that addresses societal issues. EURAM provides an opportunity to discuss and debate scientific issues in health services research as well as to present scholarly papers. This GHMFF initiative with EURAM was led by Dr. Robert Hernandez of the University of Alabama at Birmingham, who felt that faculty members should become more engaged in Europe. The first GHMFF participation was with the EURAM conference in 2008. GHMFF members then presented manuscripts at the 2009 EURAM Conference that was held in Liverpool, England. Other initiatives included presentations in the public and nonprofit management strategic interest group, a part of EURAM, in Rome, Italy; Talon, Estonia; Istanbul, Turkey; Valencia, Spain; Warsaw, Poland; Paris, France; and Glasgow, Scotland. Currently, approximately six to eight AUPHA faculty submit manuscripts that are peer reviewed and presented at the EURAM annual meeting each year.

The International Hospital Federation

The International Hospital Federation (IHF) is a not-for-profit nongovernmental organization based in Geneva, Switzerland. The IHF's vision is to create healthy communities around the world and to ensure that hospitals are efficient and well managed and provide high-quality, accessible, and patient-centered care. The IHF sponsors the World Hospital Congress, which is hosted by national hospital associations in different countries every year; sponsors an online interactive exchange platform with special interest groups (SIGs); and publishes a quarterly journal and other reports (IHF, 2017).

AUPHA has been a member of IHF since 1968 and through the years has participated in several joint projects and collaborative initiatives. In recent years the GHMFF has partnered with IHF in several activities. The Healthcare Management SIG works to advance professionalization of healthcare management globally and supports the Global Competency Directory delineating the core healthcare management competencies required for healthcare leaders globally (IHF, 2016). The Healthcare Management SIG has two main goals: to promote the professionalization of health management disciplines, and to build global capacity in the leadership and management of health systems. The IHF Healthcare Management SIG held a workshop in Washington, DC, on February 2–3, 2017. AUPHA's partnership with the IHF SIG has also resulted in the participation of the Commission on Accreditation of Healthcare Management Education (CAHME). Building on the work of the Global Consortium for Healthcare Management, during the 2017 workshop the Healthcare Management SIG members reviewed the work plan to further advance this global initiative. This SIG will focus on advancing healthcare management system improvements to achieve value-added patient care; stimulate the collaboration with academic centers and accrediting bodies; promote and support emerging hospital and healthcare management national associations; and strengthen and disseminate the healthcare management profession around the world. The development of the relationship between IHF and AUPHA through the Global Management Faculty Network has been enhanced through the collaborative work of several faculty and programs. Members of the IHF/WHO Special Interest Group include Robert Hernandez, University of Alabama at Birmingham; Bernardo Ramirez, University of Central Florida; Daniel West, University of Scranton; William Aaronson, Temple University; and Michael Counte, St. Louis University.

CAHME and International Healthcare Management Education Accreditation

A significant reason for international health administration education programs to join or interact with AUPHA through the years has been the pursuit of excellence and academic recognition. Additionally, in recent years globalization has reinforced the idea that accreditation is an important requirement to demonstrate quality.

To explore this issue, the Aramark Charitable Fund, through the Vanguard Charitable Endowment Program, provided funding to CAHME for surveying accredited programs and their faculties to understand their involvement in international health administration education (West, Filerman, Ramirez, & Steinkogler, 2011). The study started by developing an international health management education survey that sought data on demographic information, international involvement, international courses and curriculum, alumni, and ideas/opinions on global healthcare management education. The international methodology applied in this study included numerous interviews with experts on global healthcare management education. The results from the Phase I Study can be found at https://cahme.org/files/CAHME-I-Final-Report-International.pdf. Overall, the survey results showed that CAHME-accredited AUPHA graduate programs have a strong international focus in the form of study abroad, student exchanges, faculty exchanges, research, online graduate courses, and service learning abroad.

The Phase I Study also provided comprehensive information on specific programs in the following 16 countries: Australia, Brazil, Chile, China, France, India, Israel, Mexico, Philippines, Saudi Arabia, Singapore, South Africa, Spain, Sweden, Turkey, and the United Kingdom. The Phase I Study revealed that there is some, and perhaps growing, influence on health administration education by accreditation programs in business, public health, and medicine. Countries around the world are embracing accreditation standards to improve quality of care, patient satisfaction, and access to care. Many of the countries have standards that appear to be predominantly national in orientation.

The CAHME Phase II Study on International Healthcare Management Education was conducted by the same team of investigators (West, Filerman, Ramirez, & Steinkogler, 2012). The Phase II Study was made possible through a grant from the Aramark Charitable Fund. The Phase I Study showed that the health administration education system is closely articulated with the recognized needs of the healthcare delivery system in several countries. The Phase II Study utilized the existing findings from the Phase I Study but added six additional countries, including Germany, Ireland, Czech Republic, South Korea, Netherlands, and Colombia, bringing the total number of countries studied to 22. The second phase research study supported the need for some form of accreditation, whether international or national in orientation. The Phase II Study also clearly identified organizations in business, public health, and medicine that may have an interest in accreditation/certification in the sphere of influence of health services administration. The Phase II Study found that 69% of graduate programs had faculty involved with some type of international research, 42% of the respondent programs were offering study abroad, and the majority of programs (82%) used elective courses to offer study abroad. Global health management courses were offered by 38% of the CAHME programs, while 46% of AUPHA graduate programs reported having international partnerships with another country.

AUPHA Activities in Support of Membership Programs and Faculty

The AUPHA and AIHA partnership profoundly affected many faculty members' careers and awakened an interest in global programs among AUPHA member programs. AUPHA recognized this growing trend, and its Office of International Programs was instrumental in establishing the International Health Faculty Forum.

Despite the success of the Office of International Programs, a growing paucity of resources forced AUPHA to discontinue the office in 1999, as it shifted the focus to faculty-initiated activities. At the same time, faculty in many programs had been pursuing global interests through personal or university affiliations. During 2012 and 2013, Lydia Middleton (Reed) conducted two international one-week study tours for AUPHA faculty interested in expanding their global knowledge. The first one was to the Netherlands and the second one to London, to learn about the Dutch and UK healthcare systems and management education experiences and trends.

Global Health Management Faculty Forum

With the growing recognition of the impact of globalization on healthcare in the United States and elsewhere, the faculty forum rebranded itself as the GHMFF and quickly became one of the most active forums within AUPHA (Aaronson, Counte, Ramirez, & West, 2010).

The GHMFF represents a group of AUPHA faculty that has a strong interest in internationalization and globalization. The global faculty management network has been successful in building international involvement. The GHMFF's initial efforts focused on competencies in graduate health management programs. Several articles authored by GHMFF members appeared in the *Journal of Health Administration Education* addressing interests related to competency mapping, epidemiology, health literacy, diversity, developing physician leaders, environmental stewardship, and so forth.

One study within the context of the GHMFF focused on AUPHA program director perceptions of global healthcare management competencies (Aaronson et al., 2008). The article analyzed a survey administered to program directors in the United States and in several programs globally. Surprisingly, the survey revealed that U.S. program directors were very much attuned to the impact of globalization on American health services organizational performance. This translated into a need for U.S. programs to focus greater effort on developing global competencies among students. The survey also showed that there is a lack of curricular support materials and expertise to meet the perceived need.

The GHMFF developed the Annual Global Health Symposium to be conducted as part of the AUPHA Annual Meeting. Lydia Middleton (Reed), as President and CEO of AUPHA, supported this idea, offering our international partners special fees for the event that included international program membership, and thus boosting the number of international members. The initial symposium was held in 2010. The focus changes each year, but the overall intent is to engage international programs previously involved with AUPHA through the Kellogg Foundation projects in South America and the AIHA/USAID projects in CEE and NIS of the former Soviet Union regions. More importantly, the symposium provides AUPHA member program faculty with a venue in which to present and discuss common interests and experiences in global health management.

The GHMFF has focused on competencies and career development strategies, using research in health management education, international accreditation, public–private partnerships in healthcare, developing advances in healthcare management education, building sustainable global partnerships, and building international networks. The sessions have recognized the values of successful university-based and community-based partnerships, identifying factors for sustainability and factors that impede their successful development. Educational sessions have focused on short-term study abroad for graduate students enrolled in CAHME-accredited programs. More recently, GHMFF efforts have included developing global regional networks through professional associations and organizations. This has resulted in initiatives to involve organizations from Europe, Asia, South America, and Australia.

Establishing Global Health Management Competencies

In recognition of the growing importance and impact of globalization on healthcare delivery (Counte, Ramirez, & Aaronson, 2011), the Global Healthcare Management Faculty Network led an effort to develop a body of knowledge for developing curricula that are global in scope. The initial work was completed by Dr. Dan Dominguez, with input from Dr. Bernardo Ramirez and Dr. Bill Aaronson. This body of knowledge has been widely circulated and serves as a foundation for the Leadership Competencies for Healthcare Services Managers (IHF, 2016), which were developed by the Global Consortium for Healthcare Management between January 2013 and June 2015. The need for professionalization of healthcare management is a global demand, and the IHF has identified six domains for competency development. The competency framework fits with the body of knowledge developed through the Global Healthcare Management Faculty Forum. The major domains that have been assembled for the IHF competency directory mirror the Healthcare Leadership Alliance competency directory and its major domains: leadership, communication and relationship management, professional and social responsibilities, health and healthcare environments, and business.

Network Framework and Model

Some faculty members from the GHMFF have examined healthcare costs and the efficacy of healthcare systems on a global scale (Aaronson et al., 2010; Counte et al., 2011). This effort also included outcomes data from the CAHME Phase I and Phase

II studies referenced earlier in this chapter. Utilizing this body of knowledge, the faculty forum identified necessary competencies for developing community assessment and collaborative partnerships. The collaborative partnerships and networks also use study abroad, faculty–student collaborative research, and service learning to implement the body of knowledge by looking at minimum and maximum competencies required across all phases of a career (West, Ramirez, & Filerman, 2015).

The network model was presented at the IHF 39th World Hospital Congress held in 2015 in Chicago, Illinois (West et al., 2015). The network model, with the IHF Global Leadership Competency Model, could serve as a basis to identify international criteria for competency. A regional network thus must place a strong emphasis on assessment and evaluation in designing a certification/ accreditation model.

The GHMFF has endorsed the creation of a Global Council on Healthcare Management Education. The council would be organized through AUPHA and also would engage CAHME. Regional network interactions (Global Network) would include AUPHA, SHAPE, EHMA, CLADEA (Latin American Council of Management Schools), and ASPHER (Association of Schools of Public Health in the European Region). International accreditation would include a joint effort by AUPHA and CAHME. Based on several requests for international accreditation, the effort to move forward with international accreditation was approved by the CAHME Board of Directors at their June meeting in 2017. The Global Council would involve additional regions in Asia and Indonesia and include regional advisers, regional conferences, and university-based partnerships.

Collaborative Study Abroad Opportunities

CAHME's Phase I and Phase II studies, described previously, found that 30% of accredited graduate programs provide study abroad for students and 33% of graduate programs have faculty exchanges abroad. Furthermore, 37% of CAHME-accredited programs have international projects, and 51% of CAHME-accredited programs are involved with international research. The studies also revealed that 82% of graduate accredited programs encourage and support faculty to present at international conferences.

The GHMFF has examined different types of graduate-level study abroad. Recently, they considered short-term study abroad that includes 10 to 14 days of travel. The study abroad would utilize competencies developed by CAHME-accredited programs and focus on the application of knowledge that was identified through the AUPHA faculty network. Faculty agree that study abroad is an important part of graduate education. The Health Administration Program of the

University of Scranton has organized and designed a short-term study abroad model that includes a pre-phase, study abroad phase, and post-phase. The types of learning experiences have been identified and assessment and evaluation tools have been suggested in the annual symposium presentations. The post-phase submission of projects includes research, presentations, debriefing sessions, research papers, oral examinations, journals, and reflection papers. For example, at the 15th Annual Conference of the European Academy of Management in Warsaw, Poland, in June 2015, Professors West, Ramirez, Costello, and Szydlowski introduced historical perspectives on global initiatives associated with AUPHA (West & Ramirez, 2016).

FUTURE DIRECTIONS

Global transformation will continue, affecting higher education and the global economy, and presenting challenges and opportunities to rethink healthcare business opportunities. The changing academic landscape reflects increased movement of students across countries and regions of the world, and acquisitions occurring under academic free trade have national and international implications that will reshape higher education globally. Joint programs of study, cross-cultural research, and new venues of collaboration will grow as global economic pressures increase.

AUPHA has started a process to assess opportunities for international certification of undergraduate programs outside the United States and Canada. The association and CAHME are also exploring the implementation of international accreditation activities through collaborative arrangements, since the operating workforce for both initiatives will come mainly from the combined membership. CAHME, at a board meeting in June 2016, adopted a strategic business initiative that will focus on international accreditation. For several years, CAHME has entertained the idea of international accreditation and expanding its influence and impact in graduate higher education. Efforts at international accreditation will necessitate changes, requiring trained faculty who understand accreditation and have international experiences that will allow for cultural adaptations and modifications. Many accredited graduate programs have relationships with universities in other countries that have expressed an interest in accreditation. The CAHME focus will be at the graduate level and involve a twinning concept where U.S. universities can help to cosponsor and work with other universities that want to pursue accreditation.

The idea of a borderless world in higher education suggests that there may be an interest in certification for undergraduate programs. With its strong membership of undergraduate programs and experience in undergraduate certification, AUPHA will determine the feasibility of certifying undergraduate programs in the global market. Therefore, it is important that CAHME and AUPHA collaborate with universities in all regions of the world. Pressures to manage healthcare costs and to improve quality of care and patient satisfaction will increase. Consequently, undergraduate and graduate programs both must produce trained healthcare managers and leaders who can succeed in a global healthcare arena where the geopolitical landscape is constantly changing. The utilization of research to improve clinical outcomes and to develop more efficient healthcare systems further supports the need for CAHME and AUPHA to work together. Both organizations are driven by faculty. As such, the GHMFF plays a strong role in establishing direction for accreditation in global healthcare management education, as well as in helping to redesign the type of competencies needed for global healthcare leadership. The global landscape in healthcare is such that mergers and acquisitions will continue, population health and value-based care will shape the market, and regulatory efforts will be directed at increasing efficiency, improving effectiveness, and delivering equitable care. CAHME and AUPHA will need to work with faculty in graduate and undergraduate programs to ensure that students are adequately prepared in the area of financial management, understand demographic changes, appreciate the importance of public–private partnerships, can manage the operational side of organizations, and have a strong appreciation for innovation.

With the emphasis on population health, healthcare leaders and governmental agencies will be promoting community engagement and a stronger accountability of governing bodies in healthcare sector reform. Collaborative efforts in the governance of population health management require that AUPHA and CAHME understand global markets and the importance of physician alignment, physician integration, and community engagement. The Council for Higher Education Accreditation emphasizes specialized accreditation in higher education in the United States. Higher education quality review has become an imperative, focusing on outcome metrics in the areas of employment, utilization of the degree, salary, satisfaction with the profession, and other quality outcome indicators. Internal and external quality review will be undertaken by organizations and agencies outside of colleges and universities. Here again, CAHME and AUPHA will need to collaborate with the professional provider community to enhance value and student outcomes in graduate and undergraduate education. They also must work with the healthcare provider community and other social agencies to understand new delivery models and determine competencies for healthcare leaders and managers. University outcomes, program-level outcomes, and student learning outcomes will be the gauges to assess higher education's effectiveness. Again, national and international accreditation are important. Students, parents, and the public are looking for colleges and universities to provide more affordable education and to improve graduate and undergraduate teaching and learning outcomes. There will be pressures to utilize technology and distance delivery to meet the needs of the public. The advancement of distance education should serve as an enhanced platform for universities to work in twining programs and to sponsor certification and accreditation for undergraduate and graduate programs in health management education.

Most of AUPHA's global activities occur through the global faculty forum and network. AUPHA also established a Global Leadership Committee (GLC) to examine trends and forces that will influence globalization, curricula, and directions for the future. Key updates brought forth through the GLC included support to continue and maintain an established committee as part of the AUPHA Board of Directors to set policy and establish global strategic initiatives. There was a strong desire on the part of AUPHA to continue with the global healthcare faculty network in advancing strategic initiatives for global health management at the annual AUPHA meeting. The global healthcare faculty network has been very successful in conducting an annual global symposium and engaging organizations outside of the United States, including SHAPE, EHMA, CLADEA, and ASPHER. AUPHA and CAHME have endorsed the involvement of faculty and programs with the IHF and participating with EURAM. IHF and EURAM organizations have developed strategic interest groups focusing on health management education research as well as the development of competencies needed to produce skilled healthcare leaders and managers who are able to adapt to constant change and the pressures of globalization.

REFERENCES

Aaronson, W. (1997). Developing health management education in central and eastern Europe. *Journal of Health Administration Education*, *15*(3), 165–181.

Aaronson, W., Counte, M., & Ramirez, B. (2008). A comparative perspective on contemporary trends in global healthcare management education. *Journal of Health Administration Education*, *25*(2), 175–190.

Aaronson, W., Counte, M., Ramirez, B., & West, D. (2010). Global health management education: Challenges and opportunities for academic programs. *Journal of Health Administration Education*, *27*(3), 323–325.

Aaronson, W. E., & West, D. J. (1997). Health management education and development: Partnerships in central and eastern Europe, Part I. *Journal of Health Administration Education*, *15*(3), 159–164.

Aaronson, W. E., & West, D. J. (1998). Health management education and development: Partnerships in central and eastern Europe, Part II. *Journal of Health Administration Education*, *16*(2), 109–123.

Aaronson, W., West, D., Heshmat, S., & Ramirez, B. (1998). The pillars of health management education: Lessons from the CEE experience. *Journal of Health Administration Education, 16*(2), 125–144.

American International Health Alliance. (1994). I wanted to get involved. *CommonHealth*, February/March, 4–15.

American International Health Alliance. (1996). Archives of the *CommonHealth* publication. Retrieved from http://www.aiha.com/wp-content/uploads/2015/07/15-NIS-Women-Managers-Video-Debuts-in-Iowa.pdf

American International Health Alliance. (2017). History and mission. Retrieved from http://www.aiha.com/ourstory/history/

Association of University Programs in Health Administration. (1964). Minutes of Biennial Review Committee meeting and interim meeting of August 22–25. Retrieved from http://www.aupha.org/

Association of University Programs in Health Administration. (1965a). Minutes of annual meeting of May 10–12, Cornell University, Ithaca, NY. Retrieved from http://www.aupha.org/

Association of University Programs in Health Administration. (1965b). Minutes of the Executive Committee meeting of August 4, Chicago, IL. Retrieved from http://www.aupha.org/

Association of University Programs in Health Administration. (1966a). Minutes of the Executive Committee meeting of March 5, Chicago, IL. Retrieved from http://www.aupha.org/

Association of University Programs in Health Administration. (1966b). Minutes of 1966 annual meeting of April 17–20, Duke University, Durham, NC. Retrieved from http://www.aupha.org/

Association of University Programs in Health Administration. (1966c). Proceedings of the 1st Latin American Conference on Education in Hospital Administration of August 22–24, Bogota, Colombia. Retrieved from http://www.aupha.org/

Association of University Programs in Health Administration. (1967). Minutes of the 1967 annual meeting of April 16–19. Retrieved from http://www.aupha.org/

Association of University Programs in Health Administration. (1972). Institute for European Health Services Research. Program notes 49. Retrieved from http://www.aupha.org/

Association of University Programs in Health Administration. (1975). Health services organization in Finland. Faculty Institute Series. Retrieved from http://www.aupha.org/

Association of University Programs in Health Administration. (1981). Highlights of the proceedings of the First International Course on Education for Health Services Administration. Retrieved from http://www.aupha.org/

Association of University Programs in Health Administration. (1985). AUPHA Latin American Development Program. Staff report on education for health administration. Retrieved from http://www.aupha.org/

Association of University Programs in Health Administration. (1986). Staff report on education for health administration. Retrieved from http://www.aupha.org/

Association of University Programs in Health Administration. (1989, January 10). Boletin Latinoamericano de Educación en Administración de Salud [Latin American bulletin on education in health administration].

Association of University Programs in Health Administration. (1992). Staff report on education for health administration. Retrieved from http://www.aupha.org/

Association of University Programs in Health Administration. (1998). *1998 The Year in Review*. Arlington, VA: Author.

Breindel, C. (1994). AUPHA project conducts management workshop in L'Viv, Ukraine. *CommonHealth*. Retrieved from http://www.aiha.com/

Counte, M., Aaronson, W. E., & Ramirez, B. (2001). International health services management education: An overview of major efforts and lessons learned during the 1990s. *Journal of Health Administration Education*, *18*(4), 1–18.

Counte, M., Ramirez, B., & Aaronson, W. (2011). Global health management education: Essential competencies and major curricular challenges. *Journal of Health Administration Education*, *28*(2), 227–236.

DeVries, R., Kisil, M., & Ramirez, B. (1988). Education for health administration in Latin America and the Caribbean. *Journal of Health Administration Education*, *6*(4), Part II, 919–946.

European Health Management Association. (1990). Health services management education development and research: A directory of the membership (3rd ed.). Retrieved from http://ehma.org/about/

Grant, C. (1991). Accreditation, evaluation and review in Australian programs: The end of the beginning? *Journal of Health Administration Education*, *9*(2), 181–190.

International Hospital Federation. (2016). Leadership competencies for healthcare services managers. Retrieved from https://www.ihf-fih.org/resources/pdf/Leadership_Competencies_for_Healthcare_Services_Managers.pdf

International Hospital Federation. (2017). Healthcare management special interest groups (SIG). Retrieved from https://www.ihf-fih.org/activities?type=sig&section=healthcare-management

International Research and Exchanges Board. (2017). About us. Retrieved from https://www.irex.org/about-us#story

National School of Public Health of Portugal. (1983). The world of health services administration education: Presentations of the first international course on education for health services administration. Lisbon, Portugal: Author.

Pan American Health Organization. (n.d.). About the Pan American Health Organization. Retrieved from http://www.paho.org/hq/index.php?option=com_content&view=article&id=91&Itemid=220&lang=en

Pan American Health Organization. (1983). Meeting of the advisory committee of the health administration education program in Latin America and the Caribbean. *Journal of Health Administration Education, 1*(4), 441–449.

Ramirez, B., Perfiljeva, G., & Voronenko, Y. (1994). The AUPHA management training workshop. *CommonHealth, 2*(4), 10–11.

Ramirez, B., & Schreiber, W. (1995, Fall). The AUPHA management training workshop. *CommonHealth*, 16–17. Retrieved from http://www.aiha.com/

Roemer, M. L. (1976). *Health care systems in world perspective*. Ann Arbor, MI: Health Administration Press.

Sheiman, I. (2013). Rocky road from Semashko to a new health model. *Bulletin of the World Health Organization, 91*, 320–321. doi:10.2471/BLT.13.030513

Society of Health Administration Programs in Education. (2017). About the Society for Health Administration Programs in Education (SHAPE), Australia. Retrieved from http://www.shape.org.au/about-shape/

Taylor, R. J., & Taylor, S. B. (1994). *The AUPHA manual of health services management*. Burlington, MA: Jones & Bartlett Learning.

U.S. Agency for International Development. (2006). *Evaluation of the development impact of USAID/AIHA's health partnership program in central and eastern Europe*. Washington, DC: U.S. Government Printing Office.

U.S. Department of State. (2017). *Fulbright Scholar program history.* Retrieved from http://www.cies.org/history

Weeks, L. E. (1983). *Gary L. Filerman in first person: An oral history.* Chicago, IL: American Hospital Association.

West, D., Filerman, G., Ramirez, B., & Steinkogler, J. (2011). CAHME international healthcare management education. Retrieved from https://www.cahme.org/CAHME/CAHME_Resources/CAHME_Resources%20Reports/CAHME/Resources/CAHME_Reports.aspx?hkey=ac299497-81ef-4a5d-8cf8-0be7a45882c1

West, D., Filerman, G., Ramirez, B., & Steinkogler, J. (2012). CAHME phase II: International healthcare management education. Retrieved from https://www.cahme.org/CAHME/CAHME_Resources/CAHME_Resources%20Reports/CAHME/Resources/CAHME_Reports.aspx?hkey=ac299497-81ef-4a5d-8cf8-0be7a45882c1

West, D., & Ramirez, B. (2016). University based partnerships: Designing short term study abroad opportunities for graduate students. *Journal of Clinical Social Work and Health Interventions, 7*(4), 7–11.

West, D., Ramirez, B., & Filerman, G. (2015, October). Developing strategic initiatives to advance global healthcare management education. Paper presented at the 39th World Hospital Congress of the International Hospital Federation, Chicago, IL.

ABOUT THE AUTHORS

Bernardo Ramirez, MD, is Associate Professor and Director of Global Health Initiatives of the Department of Health Management and Informatics at the University of Central Florida, where he teaches the U.S. health system, international health systems, issues and trends in the health professions, quality improvement, and strategic planning. He has been the Director of the undergraduate and executive MHA programs. Dr. Ramirez is an experienced health services administrator in public and private health organizations, with experience ranging from the hospital departmental level to planning and policy. He has provided technical assistance, developed research, and conducted training for 40 years in more than 60 countries. He has been staff and a Board member of AUPHA and serves on several committees in CAHME and the International Hospital Federation.

(continued)

ABOUT THE AUTHORS *(continued)*

William E. Aaronson, PhD, is Associate Professor and Chair of the Department of Health Services Administration and Policy in the College of Public Health at Temple University. Dr. Aaronson is a recognized leader in healthcare management education, having served as program director and department chair for CAHME accredited programs. He has worked in long-term care management, been a consultant to hospitals and long-term care organizations, and served on boards of directors for long-term and primary care organizations. Dr. Aaronson has considerable international experience, including delivery of executive training programs for health system leaders and collaborative research with local faculty in several countries. He led a USAID-funded project in Ukraine to develop community-based primary care.

Daniel J. West Jr., PhD, FACHE, is Professor and Chair of the Department of Health Administration and Human Resources at the University of Scranton. He has international faculty appointments at universities outside of the USA. He has established several university-based partnerships in other countries, including the Slovak Republic, Georgia, Mexico, and Brazil. He serves on several national boards and is actively involved with the Association of University Programs in Health Administration (AUPHA) and the Commission on Accreditation of Healthcare Management Education (CAHME). He has published extensively on healthcare leadership and management and serves on numerous editorial committees. Each year, Dr. West conducts study abroad courses for graduate MHA students in European and South American countries.

CHAPTER 8

The Dissemination of Knowledge and Best Practices

Dean G. Smith, PhD

INTRODUCTION

Learning and innovation rank among the five core values of the Association of University Programs in Health Administration (AUPHA, 2016). The articulation of these core values is a relatively recent statement of long-standing beliefs that underlie AUPHA's mission and vision. The "learning value" involves sharing knowledge to foster the development of pedagogy and to improve teaching and practice. The "innovation value" includes dissemination of best practices in healthcare management and policy education. Actions taken to disseminate knowledge and best practices include both personal connections—fostered through AUPHA meetings, events, and social media—and written materials. Written materials include books, produced in cooperation with Health Administration Press, as well as the *Journal of Health Administration Education (JHAE)*. AUPHA's dissemination of knowledge and best practices in health administration education through written materials is the focus of this chapter.

HEALTH ADMINISTRATION BOOKS

The history of publishing books related to health administration education predates AUPHA by at least 180 years (e.g., Foster, 1768), and early hospital management textbooks predate the association by at least 35 years (e.g., Hornsby & Schmidt, 1913; Ochsner & Sturm, 1909). When AUPHA was founded, there were a few health administration textbooks, some written by faculty in member programs (e.g., MacEachern, 1940). Then, as now, a common topic for discussion among faculty was the content and quality of available textbooks for their classes.

During the 1960s, the W.K. Kellogg Foundation supported a series of studies published as monographs by the University of Michigan's Bureau of Hospital Administration, which had also started publishing textbooks (e.g., Berman & Weeks, 1971). Recognizing the needs of AUPHA members and the market opportunity associated with a growing field, Health Administration Press (HAP) was launched on the University of Michigan campus in 1972—with financial support from the Kellogg Foundation and cooperation of AUPHA. The first two books published by HAP were Clipson and Wehrer's *Planning for Cardiac Care* (1973) and Flook and Sanazaro's *Health Services Research and R&D in Perspective* (1973). These were considered excellent texts. *Planning for Cardiac Care* won First Award for Applied Research by *Progressive Architecture Magazine* in January 1975. The backlist of HAP publications incorporates many of the Bureau of Hospital Administration's monographs dating back to 1961 (Hess, 1961).

HAP was sold to the American College of Healthcare Executives (ACHE) in 1986 and moved to Chicago in 1996. AUPHA remains involved with HAP through a collaboration to publish textbooks under the AUPHA/HAP imprint. AUPHA also appoints members to the Editorial Board for Graduate Studies and the Editorial Board for Undergraduate Studies. HAP currently lists more than 200 books, most of which serve as textbooks.

Although there is a special relationship between AUPHA and HAP, several other companies also publish health administration textbooks, including Jossey-Bass and Jones & Bartlett Learning.

Ensuring a wide selection of textbooks is a benefit that AUPHA provides its members. This effort is managed through close partnerships and does not require the association to own the process.

MAGAZINES AND JOURNALS

Magazines, generally aimed at practitioners, and journals, generally aimed at academicians, are key means of knowledge dissemination. Health administration magazines have been in print for more than a century. *National Hospital and Sanitarium Record* (later, *National Hospital Record*) was founded in 1897. Wrote editor E. B. Smith, "No other journal on the continent has ever undertaken the class of work which will be produced in these columns, although positively of interest to the medical professions generally and especially to those engaged in hospital organization and management" (Smith, 1898). In 1913, the title was changed to *Modern Hospital*, and later the publication was split into *Modern Healthcare (Short-Term Care)* and *Modern Healthcare (Long-Term Care)*. Crain Publishing Company launched a competing magazine in 1916, *Hospital Management*, and sold it in 1952. In 1976,

Crain Communications Inc. reentered the field by purchasing and combining the two *Modern Healthcare* publications from McGraw-Hill. It continues to be a leading magazine in the field.

The American Hospital Association created *The Bulletin of the American Hospital Association* magazine in 1927, changing its name to *Hospitals* in 1936 and to *Hospitals & Health Networks* in 1993. *Hospital Management*, *Modern Hospital*, and *Hospitals* all published articles for hospital executives on new ideas and best practices in hospital management, many of which suggested the need for more training for executives.

Journals in fields closely related to health administration education have long published articles suggesting that health administration is sufficiently unique to justify research and training (Kolesar, 1959; Lentz, 1957; Munger, 1947). As stated by Goldwater (1920, p. 277) and echoed by Thompson (1983), "Like all important teaching centers, the school for hospital superintendents, yet to be established, will accomplish its most important results in the field of research."

Early research journals in healthcare management include

♦ *Inquiry: A Journal of Medical Care, Organization, Provision and Financing*, and
♦ *HSR: Health Services Research*.

Inquiry was founded by the Blue Cross Association, Division of Research, and later transferred to Blue Cross and Blue Shield of the Rochester Area, and then to Excellus Health Plan, Inc., and now to Sage Publications, Inc.

HSR is published by the American Hospital Association Health Research & Educational Trust. William S. Spector was the founding editor, and the first article was by Hess and Srikantan (1966). Yes, Irene Hess was the author of HAP's first monograph. Reflecting AUPHA's relationship with the Health Research & Educational Trust, AUPHA was permitted to appoint a co-chair of the editorial board (Filerman, 1984).

Inquiry has focused on the financing side of healthcare, and *HSR* has focused on the delivery side, with both offering compelling research.

Research-oriented journals with a greater emphasis on the healthcare manager's role include *Hospital & Health Services Administration* and *Health Care Management Review*. *Hospital & Health Services Administration*, published by the American College of Hospital Administrators (since 1976), changed its name to the *Journal of Healthcare Management* after the college changed its name to the American College of Healthcare Executives.

Health Care Management Review, published by Aspen (also since 1976), was originally edited at the Harvard School of Public Health. These journals and others offer compelling research that suggests what healthcare managers should know and, in turn, what programs in health administration might emphasize in coursework.

For many academic disciplines (e.g., economics and sociology), the relevant trade association has initiated research-oriented journals (e.g., *American Economic Review* and *American Sociological Review*) and education-oriented journals (e.g., *Economic Education* and *Teaching Sociology*), with varying levels of association involvement in the journals' ownership and operations. As with the publication of health administration textbooks, the publication of research-oriented journals on healthcare financing, delivery, and the role of management is important to the success of faculty in health administration programs. However, unlike other academic disciplines, it has not been a priority of AUPHA to own the process.

JOURNAL OF HEALTH ADMINISTRATION EDUCATION

Recognizing that health administration magazines focused on news and pragmatic issues affecting executives—and that the established journals focused on research issues for faculty—AUPHA decided that a new journal was required that would focus on education. As noted by Filerman and Austin (1983), the health administration education literature was slim and widely dispersed. AUPHA membership had grown to the point where it could support a journal in terms of both content and distribution. The thought was that a journal dedicated to health administration education could encourage scholarship on pedagogy. Beyond the market and content motivations were three organizational drivers for creating *JHAE*.

- First, having a dedicated journal helped to define the field of health administration as distinct from public administration and business administration.
- Second, publishing *JHAE* offered something tangible that program directors could use at their universities to demonstrate the academic richness of their programs. AUPHA had published a series of *Program Notes* (e.g., White, 1975) that contained research on health administration education, but these were not in a format that would command the same academic respect as a peer-reviewed journal.
- Third, the process of writing, editing, and reviewing *JHAE* brought AUPHA members together around a common activity. A number of associate editors and a broad range of editorial board members and reviewers ensured the visibility of the magazine.

Gary L. Filerman, PhD, was *JHAE*'s founding editor for issues 1(1) 1983 through 10(4) 1992. The founding editorial board included 13 U.S. faculty, 6 international representatives, and 5 practitioner representatives. Charles J. Austin served as chairman. The following people comprised the rest of the editorial team:

- Marcia S. Lane, Managing Editor
- Lydia C. Clary, Book Review Coordinator
- Douglas A. Conrad, Contributing Editor, Health Services Research
- Jeptha W. Dalston, Contributing Editor, Management Practice
- Bernardo Ramirez, Contributing Editor, La Revista de Educación en Administración de Salud
- James D. Suver, Contributing Editor, Software Review

In 1991, Donna F. Royston replaced Ms. Lane as Managing Editor.

There was much variety in the content and style of *JHAE*'s early issues. After an opening editorial by Filerman and Austin (1983), Paul Nutt (1983) provided an essay on teaching planning, John Griffith (1983) provided an essay on teaching hospital administration ("The Proper Way to Live"), and Michel Ibrahim (1983) provided an essay on teaching epidemiology. This was a great start.

Over the years, *JHAE*'s content has always reflected issues facing health administration education and AUPHA. Highlights of the initial issues include the following:

- Reflecting the association's international aspirations, the first issue included a Transatlantic Perspective (Kolderie, 1983).
- Many articles in the early years were translated into Spanish by Bernardo Ramirez.
- Reflecting AUPHA's growing interest in undergraduate education, the first issue included a Reports and Statistics article about employment of undergraduate students (Tourigny, 1983).
- In a variety of issues, Doug Conrad included abstracts from health services research publications.

In 1992, Edgar Borgenhammar joined *JHAE* as Contributing Editor for European Literature.

The *Journal* has also served as the dissemination vehicle for important addresses to the AUPHA community. The Baxter International Foundation Prize address (now the William B. Graham Prize address), the Andrew Pattullo Lecture, HCA Forum, Studer Group Forum proceedings, and similar features appear at least annually.

Stephen F. Loebs was the second editor, for issues 11(1) 1993 through 15(4) 1997, continuing with most of the original features. More than 25 papers were published on international health management education over his tenure along with a symposium on quality (Dornblaser, 1995). During this time, the Spanish translations ended, as did the contributing editor positions related to health services research, management practice, and software review. The development of electronic libraries and searches displaced the publication of abstracts and reviews. Along these same lines, early issues included reports from the AUPHA Board of Directors (Holmberg, 1983) that would later be replaced by electronic newsletters and the *AUPHA Exchange*.

Stewart B. Boxerman was the third editor, for issues 16(1) 1998 through 19(4) 2001. The biggest concern for AUPHA during this time was well documented in *JHAE*. The Proceedings of the National Summit on the Future of Education and Practice in Health Management and Policy, February 8–9, 2001, were published for all to see and comment upon (Griffith, 2001). Also in 2001, *JHAE* published its first Special Issue on the State of Online Education in Health Administration, a theme that has generated considerable scholarship over the years, including a second Special Online Education Issue in 2015.

William E. Welton was the fourth editor, for issues 20(1) 2002 through 24(3) 2007. By this time, Lydia Middleton (Reed) had become the managing editor, and *JHAE* was moving toward an online manuscript management system and the use of standardized manuscript review forms. The editorial board had expanded to include 60 persons who completed most of the manuscript reviews—all of these board members were U.S. health administration faculty. The online manuscript management system permitted access to a number of additional potential reviewers and a reduction in the size of the editorial board. The biggest issue for AUPHA during this time was the release of the Final Report of the Blue Ribbon Task Force on Accreditation (Leatt et al., 2004). Guest editors Diana Hilberman and Claudia Campbell compiled 10 articles, commentaries, and studies surrounding the Blue Ribbon Task Force report. This report changed the Accrediting Commission on Education for Health Services Administration (ACEHSA) under AUPHA into the independent Commission on Accreditation of Healthcare Management Education (CAHME). See Chapter 4 for more information.

S. Robert Hernandez and Richard Shewchuk were the fifth and sixth co-editors, for issues 24(4) 2007 through 30(2) 2013. New features added during their tenure included sections on *Teaching Tips and Tools* and *Program Management Issues*. While many prior articles fell under these themes, making these features explicit and regular increased the number of submissions to *JHAE*.

The biggest issue for *JHAE* during this time was the move from a print journal to an online resource in 2008. Due to the substantial cost for production and mailing, the AUPHA Board deliberated over the value proposition of maintaining a print journal and decided to move online. Only a few special issues of *JHAE* have been printed in limited runs for participants and other interested parties since 2008. With the movement of most journals to at least an online option, this decision has not likely adversely affected the AUPHA membership's reading of *JHAE*.

Dean G. Smith is the seventh editor, for issues 30(3) 2013 through 36(2) 2019. Three themes describe current initiatives/challenges for the journal: numbers of articles, article recognition, and topics.

With the online publication of *JHAE*, there is a much lower marginal cost per page, so the target number of pages per volume has increased from 350 to 700, subject to having an acceptable number of good quality manuscripts. With a fairly constant number of pages per article, the corresponding number of articles in the journal has also doubled. Processing a larger number of manuscripts requires more reviewers. In *JHAE*'s first year, the editor thanked 39 reviewers for their service. In the most recent year, the number of persons providing reviews exceeded 100 from a reviewer panel of more than 600 faculty and healthcare executives. To keep pace with the review process, an even larger number of reviewers and a more diverse panel is required (Smith, 2016).

The availability of *JHAE* only to member programs through a password-protected website, as well as the loss of Medline abstracting, has limited the non-AUPHA audience. The *Journal* has two ISSNs: 0735-6722 (print and linking) and 2158-8236 (electronic). Medline/Pubmed indexing includes only the print ISSN, as there was a substantial formatting process associated with creating the files for the electronic version in 2008. There are ongoing efforts to increase the visibility of articles by expanding the availability of abstracts and indexing. Applications are under consideration by Medline, Thomson Reuters, and other indexing firms. Abstracts and citations are currently available on Google Scholar, though the search engine lacks a standard citation index.

In most volumes, *JHAE* has focused on the art and science of health administration education. Special issues have occasionally included research-oriented articles (e.g., Diana, Walker, & Mora, 2015). Recognizing that health administration faculty are expected to make contributions in teaching, research, and service, the AUPHA Board of Directors has asked *JHAE* to include more articles on health services/healthcare management research. Research-oriented papers must include some reference to the value of the results for health administration education. Encouraging high-quality submissions for a nontraditional research outlet is an editorial challenge.

GOING FORWARD

AUPHA's success in fostering excellence and innovation in health management, policy education, and scholarship comes, in part, from the dissemination of knowledge and best practices in health administration education via written materials.

Through facilitation of textbook assessment and production, and direct publication of *JHAE*, AUPHA moves the field forward.

The *Journal* effectively leads the way in sharing critical information with members. The association website states that "as one of the only professional publications in the field, the *Journal* sets a standard in health administration education research." A survey of health management faculty suggests that this self-description is reasonable (Menachemi, Hogan, & DelliFraine, 2015). The *Journal* was assessed as one of the top 10 journals in the field, and in the top five among faculty with a self-identified expertise in strategic management.

In addition to the current challenges of managing more articles, increasing article visibility, and expanding coverage of health services/healthcare management research, other challenges are certain to arise. As noted by Filerman and Austin (1983, p. 2), "The journal will change over time, just as health administration practice and education changes." In keeping with its core values, AUPHA will endeavor to maintain *JHAE* as a means of written dissemination of knowledge and best practices.

REFERENCES

Association of University Programs in Health Administration. (2016). Who we are. Retrieved from http://www.aupha.org/about/visionmissionvalues

Berman, H. J., & Weeks, L. E. (1971). *The financial management of hospitals*. Ann Arbor, MI: Bureau of Hospital Administration, School of Public Health, University of Michigan.

Clipson, C. W., & Wehrer, J. J. (1973). *Planning for cardiac care: A guide to the planning and design of cardiac care facilities*. Ann Arbor, MI: Health Administration Press.

Diana, M. L., Walker, D., & Mora, A. (2015). Vertical integration strategies in health care organizations. *Journal of Health Administration Education, 32*(2), 223–244.

Dornblaser, B. M. (1995). Symposium proceedings: Educating for quality services management. *Journal of Health Administration Education, 13*(1), 183–196.

Filerman, G. L. (1984). Shared progress, issues, and responsibilities. *Journal of Health Administration Education, 2*(3), 371–383.

Filerman, G. L., & Austin, C. J. (1983). The role of the *Journal of Health Administration Education. Journal of Health Administration Education, 1*(1), 1–2.

Flook, E. E., & Sanazaro, P. J. (1973). *Health services research and R & D in perspective.* Ann Arbor, MI: Health Administration Press.

Foster, E. (1768). *An essay on hospitals, or, succinct directions for the situation, construction, & administration of country hospitals.* Dublin, Ireland: W.G. Jones.

Goldwater, S. S. (1920). The training of hospital superintendents. *National Hospital Record, 14*(4), 275–277.

Griffith, J. R. (1983). The proper way to live: Remarks on the teaching of hospital administration. *Journal of Health Administration Education, 1*(1), 27–36.

Griffith, J. R. (2001). Report of the National Summit on the Future of Education and Practice in Health Management and Policy. *Journal of Health Administration Education,* Special Issue (Fall), 5–18.

Hess, I. (1961). *Probability sampling of hospitals and patients.* Ann Arbor, MI: Bureau of Hospital Administration, School of Public Health, University of Michigan.

Hess, I., & Srikantan, K. S. (1966). Some aspects of the probability sampling technique of controlled selection. *Health Services Research, 1*(1), 8–52.

Holmberg, R. H. (1983). Report of the Board of Directors, AUPHA. *Journal of Health Administration Education, 1*(3), 327–335.

Hornsby, J. A., & Schmidt, R. E. (1913). *The modern hospital: Its inspiration, its architecture, its equipment, its operation.* Philadelphia, PA: W.B. Saunders Company.

Ibrahim, M. A. (1983). Epidemiology: Application to health services. *Journal of Health Administration Education, 1*(1), 37–69.

Kolderie, T. (1983). Government in the eighties: Shifting roles and responsibilities. *Journal of Health Administration Education, 1*(1), 91–96.

Kolesar, P. (1959). A Markovian model for hospital admission scheduling. *Management Science, 16*(6), B-384.

Leatt, P., Grady, R., Begun, J. W., Hernandez, S. R., Hilberman, D. W., Leach, D. C., . . . Sinioris, M. E. (2004). The final report of the Blue Ribbon Task Force on Accreditation. *Journal of Health Administration Education, 21*(2), 121–166.

Lentz, E. M. (1957). Hospital administration—One of a species. *Administrative Science Quarterly, 1*(4), 444–463.

MacEachern, M. T. (1940). *Hospital organization and management*. Chicago, IL: Physicians' Record Company.

Menachemi, N., Hogan, T. H., & DelliFraine, J. L. (2015). Journal rankings by health management faculty members: Are there differences by rank, leadership status, or area of expertise? *Journal of Healthcare Management, 60*(1), 17–29.

Munger, C. W. (1947). An underpopulated medical specialty: Hospital administration. *Journal of the American Medical Association, 135*(17), 1168.

Nutt, P. C. (1983). On teaching planning. *Journal of Health Administration Education, 1*(1), 3–26.

Ochsner, A. J., & Sturm, M. J. (1909). *The organization, construction and management of hospitals*. Chicago, IL: Cleveland Press.

Smith, D. G. (2016). A thank you and call for peer reviewers. *Journal of Health Administration Education, 33*(3), 511–518.

Smith, E. B. (1898). Editorial jottings. *National Hospital and Sanitarium Record, 2*(4), 32.

Thompson, J. D. (1983). The role of research in health administration education. *Journal of Health Administration Education, 1*(2), 113–115.

Tourigny, A. W. (1983). Employment patterns of baccalaureate health administration program graduates. *Journal of Health Administration Education, 1*(1), 85–90.

White, D. K. (Ed.). (1975). *Education for health services administration in the United Kingdom*. Program notes, number 66. Washington, DC: Association of University Programs in Health Administration.

ABOUT THE AUTHOR

Dean G. Smith, PhD, is Dean of the Louisiana State University Health Sciences Center—New Orleans School of Public Health and Professor Emeritus of the University of Michigan Department of Health Management & Policy. He is committed to teaching, research, and service that provides a better understanding of the financial aspects of working with and working in healthcare delivery and financing organizations. He has served as Chair of the AUPHA Board of Directors and is currently Editor of the *Journal of Health Administration Education*. He received his bachelor's degree from the University of Michigan and his doctorate from Texas A&M University.

CHAPTER 9

AUPHA and the Evolution of Health Information Technology

Brian Malec, PhD

INTRODUCTION

Health information technology's evolution as it relates to healthcare administration education follows the changing roles that information technology has played in healthcare management, policy development, and service delivery. The name for this content has changed over time, ranging from management information systems (MIS) to health information management (HIM) to health information technology (HIT) to health informatics (HI). For the sake of continuity in this chapter, HIT will be used as the topic's generic name.

A BRIEF BACKGROUND

In the 1960s and 1970s, HIT was largely limited to mainframe computers housed in large hospitals' basements or data processing departments. The technology was used to process financial and administrative transactions, dealing with the vast amount of financial data on patient care and hospital operations. Smaller hospitals might have "shared" this technology and remotely processed their administrative data.

In addition to administrative tools, HIT systems emerged throughout the 1970s in areas such as pharmacy, radiology, and laboratory. These were logical places for such applications, but they weren't always integrated into other systems.

As HIT solutions evolved from mainframes to minicomputers, microcomputers, and portable devices, the capabilities also progressed to include clinical tools and even clinical decision support systems. During this time, Association of University Programs in Health Administration (AUPHA) programs began to integrate more HIT content into their curriculums. By 1990, what was then the Accrediting Commission on Education for Health Services Administration (ACEHSA) added information technology and the management of health technology to the criteria for accreditation. Topics such as information systems analysis, design and implementation, and clinical and administrative systems became parts of health administration education.

The HIT field continued to mature into what we see today, expanding into areas such as health informatics, big data, analytics, and the advancement of artificial intelligence and precision medicine. Whereas HIT used to focus solely on "how" to provide support for administrative, clinical, and operational tasks, it is now addressing the "why" questions as well. Today's health informatics and big data are helping providers dig into topics such as access, quality, and cost containment. The "how" gets you the data, and the "why" focuses on improving and advancing an organization's clinical and administrative goals.

There have been several turning points in HIT's development over the years. The following sections discuss some of these high points and their direct impact on AUPHA's HIT curriculum at the undergraduate and graduate levels. The chapter also explores technology's impact on content delivery.

INFLUENTIAL RESOURCES: 1980–2017

Many resources from a wide range of authors have contributed to the bank of teaching materials faculty use to prepare students for the technology aspects of their healthcare administration careers. Following are two of the most notable.

Information Systems for Hospital Administration

Published in 1979, the first edition of Chuck Austin's textbook was a critical resource that systematically presented the technology content needed by health administration programs (Austin, 1979). The textbook brought together many components and provided AUPHA programs with a resource around which they could design and teach the health information management and HIT curriculum. Topics covered included the following:

- General systems theory
- Information systems, analysis, design, and implementation
- Information systems in hospitals: clinical and administrative

Later editions added topics on computer hardware, software, decision support, and information's role in strategic management.

In 1997, Chuck Austin was joined by Stuart Boxerman, DSc, in authoring the fifth edition (Austin & Boxerman, 1997). This edition also added Brian Malec and Karen Wager as contributors. The book included new topics that reflected the emerging healthcare administration challenges, focusing on managed care, information networks, the Internet, and technology's impact on health administration education. In 2003, the sixth edition added topics such as e-health applications and project management and expanded others (Austin & Boxerman, 2003).

Gerald Glandon, Detlev Smaltz, and Donna Slovensky continued the series with the seventh and eighth editions, retitled *Information Systems for Healthcare Management*. The addition of topics on governance, portfolio management, government policy, and the value of information technology brought this valuable resource into the 21st century (Glandon, Smaltz, & Slovensky, 2008).

Health Care Information Systems: A Practical Approach for Health Care Management

The book's first edition in 2005, by Karen Wager, Frances Lee, and John Glaser, brought new perspectives built on a base of existing insights about healthcare information, data quality, and information regulations, laws, and standards (Wager, Lee, & Glaser, 2005). The text included a stronger emphasis on senior management's challenges around managing HIT. The fourth edition, published in 2017, provided a deeper understanding of major forces that define and shape what healthcare administration programs need to provide to their students.

THE START OF THE HIM FACULTY FORUM

Early in the 1980s, Brian Malec, Chuck Austin, and Stuart Boxerman had the idea to create a faculty forum that would bring together faculty from all over the country who taught and/or conducted research on health information management—or managed programs that taught this content. The thought was that interested faculty could share teaching content and learn from one another. As the story goes, Malec visited Gary Filerman, PhD, then CEO of AUPHA, to propose the concept. Dr. Filerman picked up the phone, called a colleague at Shared Medical Systems (SMS), and asked for a donation. SMS gave $3,000 to help fund one of the early

AUPHA Faculty Forums. The funds were used to support forum sessions at the annual meeting, bring in guest speakers, and help build an academic community.

SURVEYING THE FACULTY

In 1984 and 1985, Brian Malec conducted two surveys of AUPHA graduate and undergraduate program faculty to get an overview of the status of information systems education. In particular, he wanted to know if AUPHA programs required health information management content, if this topic was covered in elective courses, and who was teaching those courses. The results were presented at AUPHA's 1985 Annual Meeting.

The survey revealed rich variation in how AUPHA programs approached information systems education, with differences related to meaning, interpretation, and education delivery. The following is a summary of the 1985 survey:

- Many programs, rather than offering a stand-alone course, used an integrated approach. Either by accident or design, they integrated the HIT content across several courses to cover a range of topics, such as system selection and implementation and health technology management.
- There was no clear definition of key terms, such as management information systems (MIS), hospital, hospital information systems (HIS), and health information management (HIM). Programs varied in the approach they took to teaching these concepts.
- The study showed four distinct curriculum approaches:
  - A survey course that delved into system analysis, design, and system selection
  - An operations research/quantitative methods approach to information systems
  - An MBA-level course that provided a general introduction to computer-based information systems
  - An integrated approach that spread health information management content across several courses, including finance, strategic planning, and operations research
- The survey and publication of the report was supported by a grant from SMS (Malec, 1986).

In 1988, David Zalkind and Brian Malec surveyed 1,081 alumni from 38 AUPHA graduate programs, along with a sample of AUPHA program directors, to compare and build upon the 1986 survey. The survey instrument was based on a design by Dr. Zalkind, and both Zalkind and Malec analyzed the results, which they presented at AUPHA's 1988 Annual Meeting.

Highlights of the 1988 survey include the following:

- Forty percent of alumni said they had had an introductory course in MIS in their graduate program.
- Ninety percent indicated that since graduating they had significant involvement in some aspect of MIS (computer-generated information, information system selection, and/or implementation).
- Thirty-three percent indicated that their MIS coursework did not prepare them for the "real world."
- The respondents stressed the importance of microcomputers, spreadsheets, databases, and "hands-on" student experiences.
- They indicated the need for more relevance in the curriculum, especially "real-world" examples.
- They also wanted better integration of the topic across the core and elective courses (Zalkind & Malec, 1988).

The 1986 and 1988 surveys provided a perspective on the current state of information technology education within the health administration curricula. They also revealed what was needed to better prepare students for a changing healthcare environment—one in which information is the lifeblood of effective patient care management and health services delivery. Building off these national surveys, health information faculty decided to bring the field of HIT into clearer focus. In 1988, there was discussion within the HIM Faculty Forum to develop a HIM curriculum guide. Action was taken in 1989 to move this concept forward.

A SPECIAL ISSUE AND A DYNAMIC MEETING

Under the leadership of Chuck Austin in 1989, the *Journal of Health Administration Education (JHAE)* approved a special issue with Austin and Malec as co-editors (Austin & Malec, 1990). Andersen Consulting funded the issue. Numerous meetings were held in St. Louis and Chicago to outline the publication's objectives and content. The team selected authors from across the vendor community and AUPHA program faculty. The table of contents is reprinted in this chapter's appendix. The highlights and impact of the special issue are summarized in the following list.

- HIT leaders discussed the current and future healthcare environment and the impact that information technology had and will have in the future. More specifically, discussions covered the following:
  - The evolution of high-end super computers
  - Expert systems and the future of artificial intelligence
  - The emergence of the Chief Information Officer—both the impact it had on organizational structures and the implications for health administration education
  - Health information management learning objectives for health administration programs
  - Suggestions for an ideal curriculum, assessment, and implementation strategies, and ideas for continuing education
  - Resource guide for faculty, which included a suggested bibliography and other resources

The success of the *Journal*'s special issue, along with adding information technology and management to ACEHSA's accreditation criteria in 1990, provided the foundation for a national train-the-trainer workshop. AUPHA received funding from the Pew Research Institute to create the Pew Information Management Task Force, which became the planning committee for the two-and-a-half-day workshop. IBM supported the program, which took place December 9–12, 1990, at the company's Palisades Advanced Business Institute in New York. Representatives from academia, healthcare organizations, and IBM were present, and more than 50 faculty from across the country attended.

Topics covered during the Information Management Faculty Institute included the following:

- The challenges of information management in healthcare management education
- Current and future information technologies
- Curriculum objectives design strategies and techniques
- Demonstration of IBM's advanced technology classroom
- Supporting strategic management in healthcare organizations through information management
- Information management and quality improvement
- Assessing the financial implications of information management
- The CIO: Current realities and future hopes
- The evolving role of the CIO
- Developing instructional media

In February 1991, Dr. Filerman summarized many of the outcomes from the institute in a letter to IBM's Don Hamacheck:

- Programs are beginning to update their curriculum around several dimensions:
  - Strategic planning
  - Quality management
  - Financial control
  - Information management in the organization
  - Human and organizational factors

According to Dr. Filerman's letter, he believed that the Faculty Institute at the IBM facility played an important role in helping AUPHA faculty determine what to include in information management courses in the future to better prepare students for successful careers as health services executives.

THE CHANGING CIO ROLE

In the late 1980s, when the College of Healthcare Information Management Executives (CHIME) was formed and the chief information officer (CIO) position was emerging, healthcare organizations didn't know where to find a CIO or what this kind of executive would do in the healthcare context. CIOs were common in other industries, but healthcare lagged in understanding HIT's future role and how it differed from its past—when it focused on supporting administrative tasks and not enabling clinical systems. The IT staff in healthcare organizations during the 1970s and 1980s were low-level techies who usually worked in a subbasement and reported to the finance department. The emphasis at that time was on creating cost accounting systems and addressing diagnosis-related groups and other insurance payment systems. Over time, it became evident that the HIT function was permeating organizations' strategic and operational aspects. As other industries were advancing with the use of automated systems, such as Sabre airline ticketing systems, it was clear that healthcare had fallen behind. In response, some organizations promoted their IT director, who often was good with technology but lacked strategic and leadership experience. Other organizations brought in CIOs from different industries who had no idea that physicians didn't work for the hospital and thus could not be required to adopt technology or use it. CHIME gave the healthcare CIO a professional base and provided career pathways for individuals looking to become CIOs. Boot camps and expanding professional conferences and activities brought the healthcare CIO position to what it is today.

The placement of the CIO in a healthcare organization's management structure has morphed since the early 1990s. In the past, CIOs might have reported to the chief financial officer as a nod to HIT's financial role in an organization, or the position might have reported to the chief operating officer to reflect HIT's operational impact on the delivery system. In the 21st century, it is common to have the CIO report directly to the CEO. While it used to be customary for a CIO to have a technical background, today it is more common that CIOs have clinical and managerial expertise, as their roles are less technical and more strategic (Correll & Malec, 1991).

As the 1990s progressed, AUPHA began in earnest to define what managers needed to know about the IT role and how to create organizational structures that leveraged technology to enable more efficient and effective organizations. AUPHA listened to the practitioners who wanted more HIT skills and knowledge and integrated these concepts into the curricula. The HIM Faculty Forum continued to bring information about current and evolving HIT trends to the AUPHA faculty at the association's Annual Meeting. Textbooks and research throughout the 1990s and early 2000s further expanded the knowledge base, and programs prepared healthcare leaders to have a sound basis in HIT and appreciate its importance to organizations' missions.

AUPHA AND HIMSS: PARTNERING FOR HIT EDUCATION

During 2004 to 2005, the HIM Faculty Forum began discussions with Margaret Schulte, then vice president at the Healthcare Information and Management Systems Society (HIMSS), about encouraging faculty to become more active in the annual HIMSS conference. The idea was to provide a research forum for both the AUPHA HIM Faculty Forum and the HIMSS Educator Special Interest Group, combining their talents and resources to present new practical research at the HIMSS annual conference. The result was the first Academic Forum session at the 2005 event. Since 2010, AUPHA has continued to take the lead in planning and delivering the peer-reviewed, research, half-day forum at HIMSS. More than 50 faculty have presented their practical research papers at the conference. Each year attendance has continued to expand.

HEALTH INFORMATION MANAGEMENT SYSTEM TECHNOLOGY AND ANALYSIS PROJECT

In 2005, AUPHA, in conjunction with CAHME and HIMSS, began the Health Information Management Systems Technology and Analysis Project (HIMSTA) to further assist health administration education programs in developing a robust HIT curriculum. Here is the initial charter for the work:

> The Association of University Programs in Health Administration (AUPHA), in partnership with the Commission on Accreditation of Healthcare Management Education (CAHME) and under initial major funding from HIMSS and additional financial support from Siemens, has hosted and directed the development of this curriculum for IT education in graduate programs in health administration.
>
> This curriculum is designed to support the design and delivery of a graduate level course in health information systems and technology at the graduate level. Programs and faculty have full discretion to use the entire HIMSTA curriculum as a course, or to select modules or parts of modules for classroom use. (AUPHA, n.d.a)

To begin the project, AUPHA formed a task force, led by Margaret Schulte, DBA. The members were:

- Mark Diana, PhD, Tulane University
- Kevin Leonard, PhD, University of Toronto
- Brian Malec, PhD, California State University Northridge
- David Masuda, MD, MS, University of Washington–Seattle
- Karen Wager, DBA, Medical University of South Carolina
- Kendall Cortelyou Ward, PhD, University of Central Florida
- David Wyant, PhD, Belmont University

Lydia Middleton (Reed), then President and CEO of AUPHA, and John Lloyd, former CEO of CAHME, served as valuable advisers to the project. The HIMSTA project was supported by grants from HIMSS and Siemens.

The program's first task was to explore what graduate programs were currently doing in the area of HIT education and review literature and other materials. Schulte and Malec had been creating and vetting multiple iterations of HIT competencies from 2005 to 2008. Building off these past domain models, the task force developed a set of eight major domains in which health administration graduate students should be competent. The eight domains are as follows:

- Introduction to information management
- HIT strategic planning
- Assessment, system selection, and HIT implementation
- Management of information systems and resources
- Assessment of emerging technology

- Valuation of IT to an organization
- Security and privacy
- Systems and standards

Using these domains as the foundation, the task force put out a call for authors to develop the sub-modules under each domain. Fourteen modules were created across the eight topic areas. The modules were beta tested, updated, and published in 2013. Each module contains a series of voice-over PowerPoint presentations, with a teacher's manual, exercises, exams, case studies, and other resources. All PowerPoint modules are free to the public because of the conditions in the HIMSS and Siemens grants. The teaching materials, instructor's manual, case studies, and other resources are only available to AUPHA faculty and programs. More specific information about the domains, competencies, and modules is available on AUPHA's website (AUPHA, n.d.b).

Since the modules were published in AUPHA's library, the feedback has been positive. There have been almost 900 downloads to date. Faculty have downloaded the modules, modifying them to fit their courses and generally expanding their course and program content. At present, there are no plans to update the PowerPoint modules, but the ongoing project will add new teaching resources to the library. A complete list of the contributing authors and teaching resources can be found at network.aupha.org/himstacurriculum.

LOOKING TO THE FUTURE

As a provision of the Health Information Technology for Economic and Clinical Health Act of 2009, the Office of the National Coordinator (ONC) contracted with several healthcare education programs and faculty from across the country, including faculty at AUPHA-member programs, to create modules focused on basic HIT knowledge and skills, as well as how to effectively use electronic medical records. Once completed, the government provided these modules free to educational institutions such as community colleges to develop and expand a workforce to address the growing application of healthcare IT. In 2016 and 2017, the government funded updates for many of these modules, again with numerous AUPHA faculty taking a major role. The delivery format of these new ONC-funded modules concentrated on free online six- to eight-week courses. Several educational organizations offered these courses in a cohort structure. AUPHA programs are beginning to offer or integrate these modules in undergraduate and graduate programs across the association. The following list includes a link to the home page of ONC's healthcare professional workforce training program and links to Johns Hopkins University and University of Alabama at Birmingham courses.

- ◆ ONC Curriculum Development Center
  - – https://www.healthit.gov/providers-professionals/health-it-curriculum-resources-educators
- ◆ Johns Hopkins University
  - – https://www.mnhealthit.com/act.html
- ◆ University of Alabama at Birmingham
  - – www.uab.edu/healthIT

So, what lies ahead? A survey of AUPHA programs in spring 2017 showed that we still face challenges in bringing HIT into both undergraduate and graduate education. In addition, the content is shifting as the healthcare industry moves toward value-based care, population health, electronic medical record integration, health information exchanges, big data, analytics, artificial intelligence, and other trends. How will AUPHA programs keep up with the changing competency needs? Where will programs find faculty—both full-time and adjunct—with the research knowledge, work experience, and teaching expertise to deliver the necessary depth and breadth of content?

Thomas Martin and Brian Malec presented the survey results at the 2017 AUPHA Annual Meeting. They noted that the survey revealed a number of new content areas and strategies that are not fully covered in current textbooks. For example, a few AUPHA programs are creating concentrations or certifications in areas such as data analytics, health informatics, population health, and cybersecurity. This approach could become a trend if programs are so tight with other required courses that they cannot add more courses. As a result, the concentration or certification path might expand in the future.

Content areas mentioned as essential additions to both undergraduate and graduate curricula include the following:

- ◆ Patient information privacy and security
- ◆ HIT strategies for the evolving healthcare market
- ◆ Types of healthcare data and information: clinical and administrative
- ◆ Data quality
- ◆ HIT management roles
- ◆ HIT role in population health
- ◆ HIT and health policy

Survey respondents also want to see teaching resources expand beyond textbooks and move into more case studies, simulation-based assignments, and the use of open-source technologies.

The good news is that we now have systems and technology to gather, store, and analyze data. The challenge is to convert that information into knowledge, both clinical and administrative. This leads to the next stage of big data and analytics, which will require leaders who can embrace HIT's role in achieving an organization's mission, as well as the Triple Aim of access, quality, and cost control. Although this next stage of HIT and health informatics content in health administration programs is going to be challenging, it has some truly exciting possibilities. The key will be to work together to address the hurdles while enthusiastically embracing new opportunities.

APPENDIX

Special Issue of the *Journal of Health Administration Education*: *Information Systems Education for Future Health Services Administrators* (Austin & Malec, 1990).

Table of Contents
- *Part I: IS in the 1990s and beyond: An environmental assessment*
  - *Impact of technology in health care and health administration: Hospital and alternative care delivery systems*, John K. Kerr and Richard Jelinek, PhD
  - *The environment and future of health information systems*, James B. Martin, PhD
  - *The CIO's location in the organizational structure: Implications for health administration education*, Ralph Bell, PhD, and Brian T. Malec, PhD
    - Commentary: Stuart B. Boxerman, DSc
- *Part II: IS attitudes, knowledge, and skills: Expectations, learning objectives, implementation strategies, and continuing education*
  - *Expectations and outcome skills for a generalist healthcare administrator*, V. Brewster Jones and L. Clark Taylor, Jr., PhD
  - *An ideal curriculum model*, Charles J. Austin, PhD, and Brian T. Malec, PhD
  - *IS curriculum assessment and implementation strategies*, Brian T. Malec, PhD
  - *Continuing education needs of board members, administrators and health care personnel*, Stuart Boxerman, DSc, Richard C. Peterson, and Susan Welton
- *Part III: Resources*
  - *A resource guide and practitioners*, Gloria J. Holland, PhD
  - *Select IS Bibliography*, Brian T. Malec, PhD

REFERENCES

Association of University Programs in Health Administration. (n.d.a). A curriculum for graduate education programs in health administration. Retrieved from http://network.aupha.org/himsta

Association of University Programs in Health Administration. (n.d.b). HIMSTA curriculum: Introduction and outline. Retrieved from http://network.aupha.org/viewdocument/himsta-curriculum-introduction-and-outline

Austin, C. J. (1979). *Information systems for hospital administration* (1st ed.). Chicago, IL: Health Administration Press.

Austin, C. J., & Boxerman, S. B. (1997). *Information systems for health services administration* (5th ed.). Chicago, IL: Health Administration Press.

Austin, C. J., & Boxerman, S. B. (2003). *Information systems for healthcare management* (6th ed.). Chicago, IL: Health Administration Press.

Austin, C. J., & Malec, B. T. (Eds.). (1990). Information systems education for future health services administrators. *Journal of Health Administration Education, 8*(1), 1–4.

Correll, R., & Malec, B. T. (1991). The Chief Information Officer as a new administrator. In C. A. Weaver, J. M. Kiel, M. J. Ball, J. V. Douglas, R. I. O'Desky, and J. W. Albright (Eds.), *Healthcare information management systems: A practical guide* (pp. 235–242). New York, NY: Springer-Verlag.

Glandon, G. L., Smaltz, D. H., & Slovensky, D. J. (2008). *Information systems for healthcare management* (7th ed.). Chicago, IL: Health Administration Press.

Malec, B. T. (1986). The status and diffusion of management information systems education in programs of health administration. *Journal of Health Administration Education, 4*(2), 275–281.

Wager, K. A., Lee, F. W., & Glaser, J. P. (2005). *Health care information systems: A practical approach for health care management* (1st ed.). San Francisco, CA: Jossey-Bass.

Zalkind, D. Z., & Malec, B. T. (1988). National survey of health administration program graduates on management information systems education. *Journal of Health Administration Education, 6*(2), 319–335.

ABOUT THE AUTHOR

Brian Malec, PhD, is Professor and program coordinator at the Master of Science in Health Administration program, College of Health and Human Development at California State University, Northridge. His main areas of teaching include healthcare economics and national health policy, health information systems, and quantitative decision-making. His areas of research include HIT workforce development, measuring and managing the economic value of HIT, and teaching HIT in graduate programs. Dr. Malec is a frequent presenter and/or moderator at national and international conferences including HIMSS, HIMSS Europe, and HIMSS Asia Pacific. He is also the leader of the AUPHA Academic Forum, which presents faculty research each year at HIMSS. He has recently written and edited a book on careers in health information technology.

CHAPTER 10

AUPHA and Evidence-Based Management

Anthony R. Kovner, PhD

INTRODUCTION

Evidence-based management is a process that enables better decision making through obtaining the best available evidence—scientific, organizational, or experiential—that demonstrates stakeholder impact. This is a method for making decisions via the conscientious, explicit, and judicious use of the best available evidence from multiple sources. The steps involved include the following:

- Translating a practical problem into an answerable question
- Systematically searching for and retrieving the evidence
- Critically judging the evidence's trustworthiness and relevance
- Weighing and pulling together the evidence
- Incorporating the evidence into the decision-making process
- Evaluating the outcome of any decision that is made

Evidence-based management involves applying evidence-based practice to management. The idea of applying evidence-based practice occurs in other healthcare fields as well, such as medicine, nursing, and dentistry. It also applies in other sectors, such as policing and transportation. In general, evidence-based practice leads to increased use of metrics, stronger performance measurement, greater transparency surrounding results, and more focused accountability for performance.

This chapter explores the Association of University Programs in Health Administration's (AUPHA's) relationship with evidence-based management both now and in the future.

AUPHA'S EVIDENCE-BASED MANAGEMENT WORK TO DATE

One of AUPHA's first forays into the concept of evidence-based management was led by Anthony R. Kovner, PhD, Professor Emeritus at the Wagner School of Public Service at New York University (NYU), and Lydia Middleton (Reed), then President and CEO of AUPHA.

Middleton engaged Quint Studer, then President of Studer Group, and together with co-editors David Fine, then CEO of St. Luke's Episcopal Health System in Houston, and Richard D'Aquila, Chief Operating Officer at Yale New Haven Hospital, the group co-edited *Evidence-Based Management in Healthcare*, first edition, published by Health Administration Press and AUPHA in 2009 (Kovner, Fine, & D'Aquila, 2009). In the book, the authors argued that just as getting clinical decisions right requires wide-scale application of evidence-based medicine principles, successful implementation of evidence-based medicine requires the support of evidence-based management.

Kovner and Middleton, among others, suggested that evidence-based management would be a good theme for the 2012 AUPHA Annual Meeting in Monterey, California. They organized a panel of speakers on the theme, including Tom Rundall from the University of California, San Francisco; Eric Barends, Executive Director of the Center for Evidence-Based Management; Lynn McVey, a New Jersey hospital administrator; and Kovner. At roughly the same time, an annual meeting was being held in San Francisco for the governing board of the Center for Evidence-Based Management, led by Professor Denise Rousseau of Carnegie Mellon University. Professor Rousseau participated in the AUPHA discussions as well.

AUPHA gave visibility to evidence-based management at an important time in its development. Program faculty became much more familiar with the topic than they would have been otherwise. Certain programs, such as the program at the University of Alabama at Birmingham under Bob Hernandez's leadership, soon integrated evidence-based management into their educational programs, with a particular emphasis at the PhD level. Others, such as Rush University, with its focus on integrating management with management education, used and taught evidence-based principles in its teaching and research. Andy Garman led this effort.

A second edition of the evidence-based management book was recently released. Kovner co-edited this manuscript with NYU Professor Tom D'Aunno. This edition is titled *Evidence-Based Management in Healthcare: Principles, Cases, and Perspectives* and was published by AUPHA and Health Administration Press in 2017 (Kovner & D'Aunno, 2017). Many of the authors wrote chapters for the first edition and participated in the 2013 Annual Meeting in Monterey. Additional authors and co-authors are from AUPHA program faculty or former faculty. These include the following:

- Tom D'Aunno, John Billings, and John Donnellan of NYU
- Andy Garman, Tricia Johnson, Chien-Ching Li, Shital Shah, and Peter Butler of Rush
- Kyle Grazier and John Griffith of the University of Michigan
- Joanne McGlown, Steve O'Connor, and Richard Shewchuk of the University of Alabama at Birmingham
- Larry Prybil of the University of Kentucky
- Tom Rundall of the University of California, Berkeley

Case Example of NYU Wagner

In Spring 2016 and Spring 2017, Eric Barends taught a seven-week course in evidence-based management at NYU Wagner. The syllabus is available in the Instructor's Manual for *Evidence-Based Management in Healthcare: Principles, Cases, and Perspectives*. Evidence-based management has been a central theme in the capstone courses taught for many years at NYU Wagner by Anthony Kovner and John Donnellan.

In 2016, Dean Glied and Kovner conceived a two-year program for NYU Wagner to enhance its faculty's capability to teach and do research using evidence-based practice. The two were successful in raising funds ($150,000), and the program was launched in September 2017.

Conversations about the program have centered on developing student skills and improving the delivery of critical learning outcomes. Themes include the following:

- Critical thinking (and suspicions of "facts")
- Conceptualizing data, which requires numerical fluency and intuitions about data
- Basic and intuitive understanding of probabilities
- The added value of qualitative research
- Improving capacity to learn by doing and in partnership with others
- Evaluating evidence quality from all information sources (sniffing out bad science)
- Recognizing cognitive biases
- Acknowledging that scientific evidence is relevant to management practice
- Appraising learning outcomes of all the above

(continued)

Kovner and Glied discussed a modular approach to enriching the curriculum, suggesting a toolkit version of Eric Barends's existing course with online elements and material that faculty can integrate in other courses. The university is moving ahead with a group randomized trial to evaluate the effect of evidence-based management training on capstone course performance. A first trial could measure the effect a short course about searching for peer-reviewed research might have on the quality of the literature review students conduct in the two-semester capstone course. This first trial would involve two experimental training conditions, face-to-face and online delivery, and a control.

NYU Wagner has recruited Denise Rousseau, Professor of Management at Carnegie Mellon, and Eric Barends to lead the program, spend two months a year for two years with faculty and students in New York City, and develop a research study relating skills in evidence-based management to skills required on the job.

As of early 2018, evidence-based practice is still a work in progress under the leadership of Denise Rousseau and Eric Barends, as is its usefulness and relevance for AUPHA faculty and students. The university is hopeful that results of the research and the experience will be shared with the AUPHA membership at a future annual meeting and in the AUPHA *Journal of Health Administration Education*.

THE NEXT STEPS FOR EVIDENCE-BASED MANAGEMENT

The theories and practice surrounding evidence-based management are still evolving. As such, AUPHA must remain flexible in how it approaches and incorporates this methodology. Here are some questions the association must consider in planning for the future:

- How can we influence faculty to more fully apply evidence-based practice in their teaching and research?
- Where does evidence-based management fit in the Commission on Accreditation of Healthcare Management Education–approved curriculum?
- How can we make a stronger evidence-based case for evidence-based practice?

Although this author does not presume to have the answers to these questions, they are still worth raising. AUPHA and its member programs face a challenging environment, given that U.S. healthcare costs much more than healthcare in other countries and produces no better results. Similarly, healthcare managers in the United States are more highly paid than those in other countries, and there are more of them as a percentage of the healthcare workforce. Waste is estimated at 30 percent of U.S. healthcare expenditures—much of it spent on billing and collecting for health services in payment systems, which are much more complex than need be, judging from the experience of other countries.

Proponents of evidence-based management hold that managers can make better decisions based on the highest quality evidence available, and that they can be trained to learn and practice a better decision-making process in response to sets of answerable questions, following the steps of the evidence-based management process.

Faculty Use of Evidence-Based Practice

One question that arises when considering how evidence-based practice applies to health administration education is whether students could learn more or better with the aid of evidence-based practice. In this author's experience, there is a lot of benefit in faculty working to define, assess, and respond to performance expectations. Ways to do this include the following:

- Contracting with healthcare organizations as sponsors and having the organizations present to bid contracts to the capstone class
- Spending most of the first semester of a two-semester course negotiating a contract of work with answerable questions for the client
- Reviewing the four sources of evidence—scientific literature, organizational evidence, experiential evidence, and stakeholder concerns
- Pursuing objective measurement through the process
- Holding student teams accountable for results relative to the contract objectives

The method of inquiry is emphasized in the student engagement rather than program recommendations.

Faculty can examine whether their own practices follow an evidence-based practice process. A good place to start is to focus on student assignments. One possible evidence-based assignment students could complete is assessing their own current skills and objectives in relation to the job they want to pursue after graduation. Students can then be asked to posit the skills and experience needed to get the desired job and draw up a plan for reaching the goal and overcoming constraints to implement the plan.

A faculty member should also consider whether he or she follows the steps of the evidence-based management process in designing the course syllabus and in measuring learning results, both in the classroom and after the student graduates and is on the job.

Evidence-Based Management and Required Program Curriculum

Evidence-based practice should be part of the required curriculum in all health administration programs. Students should be taught how to make decisions through the conscientious, explicit, and judicious use of the best available evidence from multiple sources. The process includes the steps of asking, acquiring, appraising, aggregating, applying, and assessing.

Teaching skills for better decision making can be implemented in three ways:

1. Add a full or half (seven-week) course in evidence-based practice.
2. Substitute the evidence-based practice course for sessions in the required organizational behavior course or in the health administration course.
3. Organize evidence-based sessions into one- to three-session modules, which can be substituted for existing sessions in these courses.

An Evidence-Based Argument for Evidence-Based Practice

Recently, an entire issue of *Health Affairs* (March 2017) was devoted to delivery system innovation where processes similar to evidence-based practice can be applied to launching and evaluating delivery system innovation. Vaida (2017) concluded, concerning new payment models tying dollars to better patient outcomes for super-utilizers of care, that

> all of the models involve expanding a patient's care from a single provider to an integrated health team. . . that includes access to behavioral health and social services such as food, housing and transportation. Often the care team will then follow up with patients repeatedly to make sure they get the care they need. (p. 394)

Vaida implies that evidence-based practice or some similar process can help show which of the promising strategies under what circumstances are most effective, in this case, for addressing super-utilizers.

Evidence-based management already drives improved organizational performance. Some major healthcare organizations, such as Kaiser Permanente and Geisinger, use evidence from operations to respond to answerable questions and stimulate management innovations. Evidence-based practice has grown in medicine and nursing. It leads to the increasing use of metrics in healthcare, measuring performance, increasing transparency of results, and providing more focused accountability for performance. The NYU Wagner current demonstration in evidence-based practice shows promise of moving in this direction.

CONCLUSION

AUPHA has played a leadership role in introducing evidence-based management to its member programs. Going forward, evidence-based practice could well be a brand for AUPHA programs, especially those that are accredited. The evidence-based framework can be applied to AUPHA as an organization as well. How are healthcare managers in the United States being educated, and how should they be? What should be the role of AUPHA and its programs in their education? This question should be systematically reviewed and addressed.

REFERENCES

Kovner, A. R., & D'Aunno, T. A. (Eds.). (2017). *Evidence-based management in healthcare: Principles, cases and perspectives* (2nd ed.). Chicago, IL: Health Administration Press.

Kovner, A. R., Fine, D. J., & D'Aquila, R. (Eds.). (2009). *Evidence-based management in healthcare*. Chicago, IL: Health Administration Press.

Vaida, B. (2017). For super-utilizers, integrated care offers a new path. *Health Affairs, 36*(3), 394–397.

ABOUT THE AUTHOR

Anthony R. Kovner, PhD, is Professor Emeritus at the Wagner School of Public Service at New York University (NYU), where he was Director of the Health Policy and Management program for 16 years. Formerly, he had been Director of the Health Services Management Program at the Wharton School of the University of Pennsylvania. He has served as a member of the AUPHA Board of Directors and as chair and member of various AUPHA committees and task forces. He has authored 11 books, co-edited textbooks, and published more than 90 peer-reviewed articles, many of them case studies. Kovner was the fourth recipient of AUPHA's Gary L. Filerman Prize for Educational Leadership.

CHAPTER 11

AUPHA Today

Gerald L. Glandon, PhD

INTRODUCTION

The 70-year history of the Association of University Programs in Health Administration (AUPHA) largely shapes its position in 2018. As an organization, AUPHA has matured from an idea originating with a handful of concerned and motivated healthcare leaders in the late 1940s to an organization that has an established reputation and a solid position in the healthcare landscape. This chapter briefly outlines the current state of AUPHA in terms of its roles and value as a national and international association of healthcare management experts united by a common mission.

VISION, MISSION, AND VALUES

Throughout AUPHA's history, the organization has crafted strategic plans to establish priorities and guide its future. The latest one began with a reconsideration of the organization's vision, mission, and values, providing direction to the AUPHA Board of Directors, staff, and membership. Over the years, the articulation of this crucial doctrine has evolved but, for the most part, stayed relatively constant. As presented in the box on page 156, the vision was unchanged from prior statements because AUPHA continues through its member organizations to develop leaders with the values and competencies necessary to drive improvement throughout the health system. These values and competencies reflect the realization that healthcare involves the public trust. Like other business leaders, those responsible for healthcare organizations must have an array of competencies; however, they must also have the values to attain and maintain public trust.

The mission statement did change significantly. After intense discussion and debate, the Board decided to include "scholarship" in the mission statement. Reinstating scholarship brings AUPHA closer to its origin. Our mission to foster excellence and innovation must include the creation of new knowledge through a commitment to scholarship.

Finally, the AUPHA Board reaffirmed the five core values that guide members and staff. Now, more than ever, excellence, innovation, collaboration, diversity, and learning establish our brand and contribute to the association's success.

AUPHA VISION

To develop leaders who possess the values and competencies necessary to drive improvement throughout the health system.

AUPHA MISSION

AUPHA fosters excellence and innovation in health management and policy education and scholarship.

AUPHA VALUES

AUPHA achieves excellence and innovation in health management and policy education and scholarship by embracing diversity and providing opportunities for learning and collaboration.

Excellence: AUPHA believes that excellence in education leads to excellence in health management practice, and ultimately leads to improved quality, efficiency, and accessibility in healthcare delivery.

Innovation: AUPHA promotes innovation, encourages the adoption of new strategies, and disseminates best practices in health management and policy education.

Collaboration: AUPHA collaborates in the generation and translation of research and the integration of theory and practice in interprofessional work environments.

Diversity: AUPHA believes diversity—in people, in programs, and in perspectives—is essential for an effective interprofessional workforce.

Learning: AUPHA pursues continual learning to advance and share knowledge, to foster the development of pedagogy, and to improve teaching and practice.

AUPHA MEMBERSHIP

Currently, AUPHA membership exists at two primary levels. The formal membership is made up of academic programs that have joined AUPHA in one of the many membership categories. In addition, the 2,400 individual faculty associated with these member programs also receive AUPHA member benefits. This dual aspect of membership makes defining AUPHA a challenge. Does it consist of dues-paying academic programs or the faculty from those member programs? AUPHA is both. Unfortunately, member programs do not necessarily list all of their faculty as being a part of the AUPHA family. Consequently, while we list a substantial portion of a program's faculty involved with preparing future leadership, we are not able to list them all.

At the end of 2017, AUPHA membership consisted of 238 programs. This number steadily increased over the last several years (see Chart 1). Of this total, 124 programs were either accredited graduate programs (by CAHME) or certified undergraduate programs. The remaining 114 were mostly associate graduate or undergraduate programs and a small number of doctoral programs.

The accredited and certified programs are called full programs because once they receive accreditation from CAHME or are certified by AUPHA, they receive full voting and other member benefits. Of the 124 full programs, 78 have CAHME accreditation and 46 have AUPHA certification. Both these numbers have stayed relatively constant in recent years, as displayed in Chart 2.

Chart 1. Accredited/Certified and Total Programs: 2010–2017

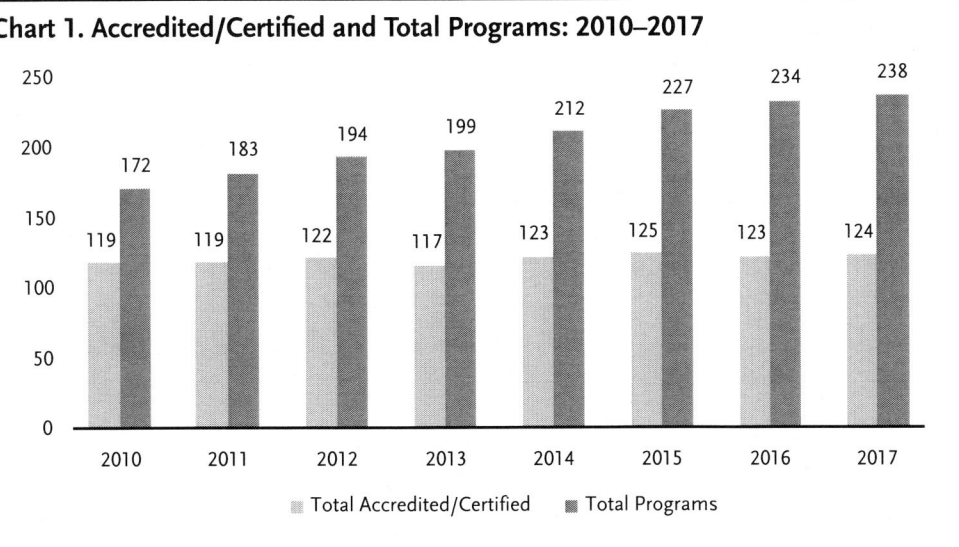

Chart 2. Full Graduate and Full Undergraduate Programs: 2010–2017

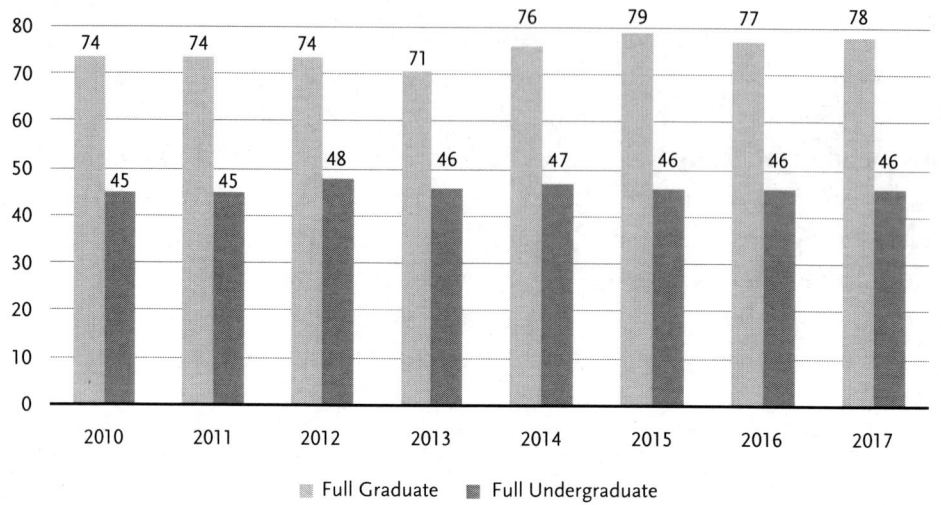

Full Graduate ▪ Full Undergraduate

As seen in Chart 3, the number of member programs that have not yet received either accreditation or certification has been growing.

Finally, Chart 4 presents the breakdown of member programs in 2017 by the type of college they reside in within their broader universities. Although "health professions and allied health" is the largest single category, AUPHA consists of programs residing in an array of other academic settings.

Chart 3. Associate Graduate and Associate Undergradute Programs: 2010–2017

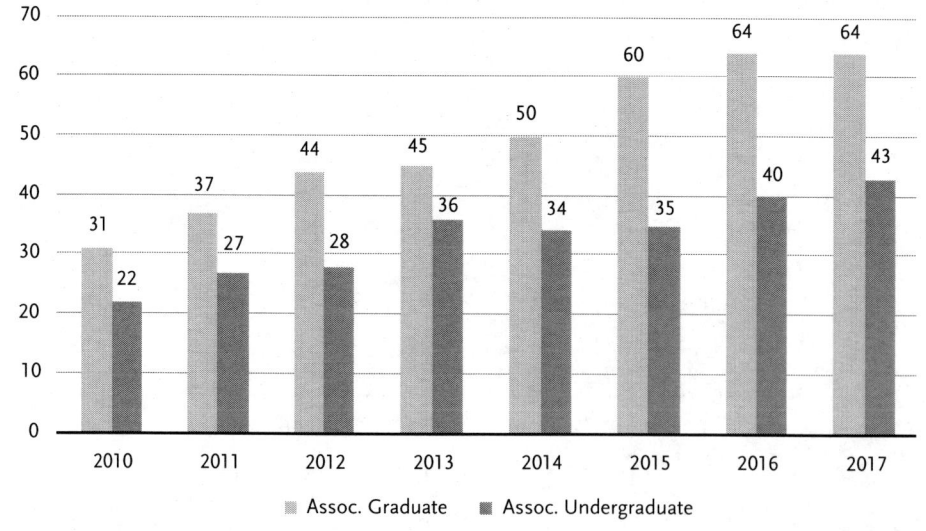

Assoc. Graduate ▪ Assoc. Undergraduate

Chart 4. Proportion of AUPHA Member Programs by College Setting: 2017

College Setting	Percent
Health Professions*	47.8
Public Health	17.0
Business	18.3
Other**	17.0

* Includes Allied Health
** Consists of nursing, medicine, graduate studies, public administration, and unclassified.

Regarding the composition of individual faculty associated with AUPHA, we get an additional sense of diversity. As Chart 5 indicates, the greatest proportion of faculty are associated with accredited graduate programs followed by associate undergraduate programs. Several considerations cloud these data, however. As mentioned before, not all faculty associated with a member program are listed as AUPHA-affiliated. In addition, a number of organizations have multiple programs as members of AUPHA. For these related programs, the assignment of faculty to graduate, undergraduate, or doctoral programs is difficult at best because many teach in all three. We let program leadership make this assignment.

There is also variance in the participating faculty's degree preparation. While most report having a PhD, a substantial number have a variety of other types of doctoral preparation (see Chart 6). Further, just under 20 percent report having an MHA, MBA, or similar master preparation. A note on these data as well. First, many faculty fail to indicate their terminal degree, so these percentages are based on only a portion of the total members in the AUPHA database. Second, a substantial

Chart 5. Percentage of Participating Faculty by Program Type: 2017

Program Type	Percentage of Faculty
Accredited Graduate	36.85
Associate Graduate	15.56
Certified Undergraduate	12.68
Associate Undergraduate	27.13
Associate Doctoral	1.44
All other*	6.18

*"All other" includes affiliate, individual, and international members.

Chart 6. Percentage of Participating Faculty by Reported Degree: 2017

Faculty Degree	Percentage
PhD	59.28
MBA/MS	18.08
MD	4.48
Nursing	2.64
DrPH	3.60
JD	4.40
EdD	3.20
Other doctoral	4.32

Note: Nursing includes all levels of nursing.

number of individuals report more than a single degree, and we only include the first degree reported in our analysis. Many nurses with PhDs, for example, report the doctoral degree first, thus underrepresenting nursing in these percentages. Also, the failure to report may be due to confusion over which degree is the most appropriate.

While other aspects of faculty diversity exist, only geographic location seems to matter further. It is interesting that faculty report living in 44 states plus Washington, DC, and Puerto Rico, along with three Canadian provinces. Florida, Texas, North Carolina, and Illinois have the most AUPHA members, corresponding generally to the overall population in those states.

FINANCIAL POSITION

AUPHA's financial position is an essential element for its ultimate success. There is no sustained ability to function long term if revenue does not exceed expenses at least most of the time. By the same token, however, because AUPHA is primarily dependent on dues for revenue, it is vital that members not endure all the financial burden associated with AUPHA operations.

Chart 7 shows AUPHA's revenue and expenses, which have not moved a great deal since 2008. For this period and much of AUPHA's existence, the generation of net income has not been a primary goal. The Board targets about three percent of operating expenses as a general goal for net income.

Chart 8 shows AUPHA's endowments and reserves from 2008 to November 2017. All of these increased substantially during the last 10 years. Note the "small

Chart 7. Total Actual Revenue, Expenses, and Net Income by Year: 2008–2017

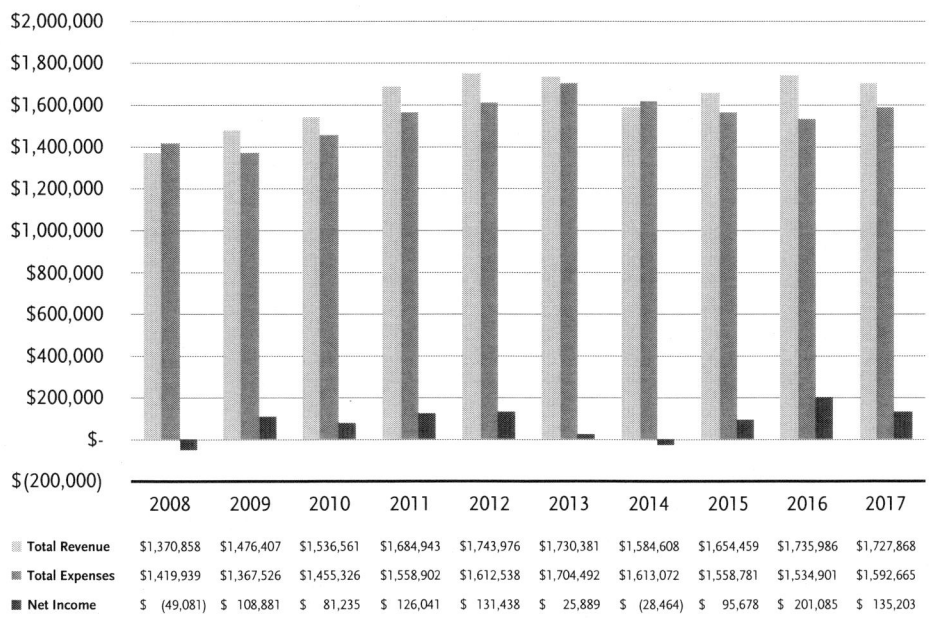

	2008	2009	2010	2011	2012	2013	2014	2015	2016	2017
Total Revenue	$1,370,858	$1,476,407	$1,536,561	$1,684,943	$1,743,976	$1,730,381	$1,584,608	$1,654,459	$1,735,986	$1,727,868
Total Expenses	$1,419,939	$1,367,526	$1,455,326	$1,558,902	$1,612,538	$1,704,492	$1,613,072	$1,558,781	$1,534,901	$1,592,665
Net Income	$ (49,081)	$ 108,881	$ 81,235	$ 126,041	$ 131,438	$ 25,889	$ (28,464)	$ 95,678	$ 201,085	$ 135,203

Chart 8. Total Endowments and Reserves by Year: 2008–2017

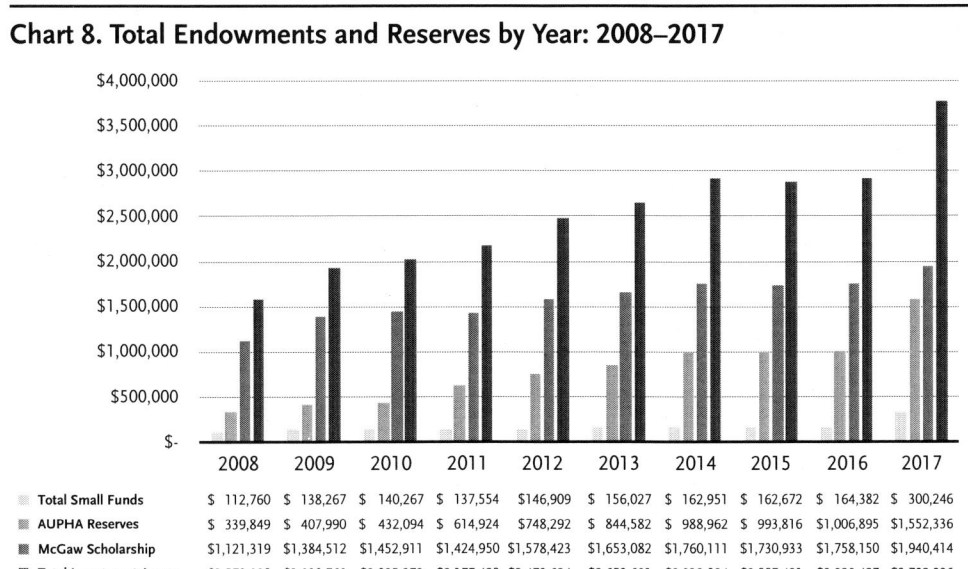

	2008	2009	2010	2011	2012	2013	2014	2015	2016	2017
Total Small Funds	$ 112,760	$ 138,267	$ 140,267	$ 137,554	$146,909	$ 156,027	$ 162,951	$ 162,672	$ 164,382	$ 300,246
AUPHA Reserves	$ 339,849	$ 407,990	$ 432,094	$ 614,924	$748,292	$ 844,582	$ 988,962	$ 993,816	$1,006,895	$1,552,336
McGaw Scholarship	$1,121,319	$1,384,512	$1,452,911	$1,424,950	$1,578,423	$1,653,082	$1,760,111	$1,730,933	$1,758,150	$1,940,414
Total Investment Assets	$1,573,928	$1,930,769	$2,025,272	$2,177,428	$2,473,624	$2,653,691	$2,912,024	$2,887,421	$2,929,427	$3,792,996

funds" item consists of the Filerman Award Fund, the Thompson Award Fund, the Pattullo Lecture Fund, and the Bachrach Scholarship Fund. These together support both students and faculty through recognition and/or cash awards.

STAFF

AUPHA's staff has evolved over the years to reflect changes in program needs and available technology. Currently, there are five salaried employees and two contracted/temporary staff.

The president and chief executive officer is responsible to the AUPHA Board of Directors for the execution of the association's strategic plan, the implementation of its programs, and the executive leadership of AUPHA's staff. The president/CEO is ultimately responsible for the association's complete operation and effective functioning. This position works with all major constituencies associated with the organization. Gerald Glandon is the current president and CEO and reports directly to the Board of Directors. Other staff include the following:

- ◆ Vice President and Chief Operating Officer
- ◆ Finance Manager
- ◆ Director of Membership
- ◆ Manager of Meetings and Services
- ◆ Consultant for Programs/Awards and Undergraduate Certification

MAJOR ACTIVITIES

AUPHA reaches out and involves its membership in several ways. The following sections take a close look at some of these endeavors.

The Faculty Forum Network

AUPHA has pursued a goal of engaging faculty members in a robust exchange of ideas through Faculty Forums and other online mechanisms. This process began in 1998 and makes it clear that AUPHA values the open sharing of ideas to further healthcare management education. The Faculty Forums arose because many individual faculty members have few colleagues in their discipline, host programs, colleges, or universities. The AUPHA Faculty Forums facilitate virtual meetings and idea sharing, fostering innovative teaching techniques, evolving content, and professional collaborations.

During its July 1998 meeting, the AUPHA Board of Directors approved parameters and guidelines for establishing the Faculty Forums:

1. The Faculty Forum is an official working group sanctioned by the AUPHA Board of Directors to facilitate faculty exchange on a regional, national, or multinational scale.
2. The Faculty Forum is topic- or issue-specific and is sanctioned for a specified duration to accomplish this objective.
3. Unlike an AUPHA Task Force, for which membership is determined by the AUPHA Chair, membership in a Faculty Forum is based exclusively upon faculty electing to participate.
4. Faculty Forums are self-governing. The AUPHA Board Chair shall appoint a convener. Any faculty member of an AUPHA member program is eligible to participate in any forum.
5. Once established, AUPHA staff will maintain a registry of all Faculty Forums, membership, and conveners. A list of forums and conveners will be published annually.
6. To establish a Faculty Forum, faculty from five different AUPHA member programs must present to the Board a petition indicating proposed purpose, tentative plans, and members.
7. The AUPHA Board will review and recertify existing forums at its summer meeting and will accept petitions for the creation of a forum at any time. Conveners of existing forums will present to the Board a written report of accomplishments, membership, participation, and future plans in May of each year.
8. AUPHA staff will ensure that every forum has the opportunity to caucus at the AUPHA Annual Meeting.
9. The AUPHA Board will decertify a forum for failure to demonstrate effective faculty exchange and/or if the forum fails to serve the corporate objectives of AUPHA.
10. AUPHA will devote available staff time to support forums based upon the decision of the President. AUPHA is not responsible for any operational costs associated with a forum.

There are currently 15 faculty forums. Here is a brief description of each.

Advancing Women Leaders in Healthcare
This forum works to identify special issues related to women in management positions. Members work collaboratively and inclusively across race, class, gender, ethnicity, sexual orientation, religion, differing abilities, generations, and so on to address concerns of women working and studying in professional and academic settings. The forum's ultimate goal is to provide necessary professional development

opportunities that advance women to higher levels of leadership in the profession. The group currently has 124 members.

Cultural Perspectives

With 91 members, this forum helps the academic community build an inclusive culture of development and productivity by providing examples of how to build higher performing organizations and the tools to do so.

Ethics

The forum provides resources for teaching ethics to health administration students, whether as a primary course or by integrating the topic into other courses. The forum facilitates the exchange of ideas, and members share best practices and collaborate to develop innovative teaching strategies. There are currently 83 members.

Finance, Economics, and Insurance

With 117 members, this forum works to identify core knowledge/skills in accounting, finance, economics, and insurance for both undergraduate and graduate programs, and develops basic competencies for accreditation.

Global Healthcare Management

The forum has the following goals: to continue the development of global healthcare management (GHM) education domains and competencies; to create communication tools and resources for the faculty forum; to share GHM syllabi and teaching resources; to explore AUPHA certification of foreign programs; and to improve teaching technology. There are currently 132 members.

Health Information Management

The forum aims to enhance the ability of undergraduate and graduate healthcare administration faculty to teach, research, and provide service in the field of healthcare information technology. It has 122 members.

Health Policy

This forum is a virtual center for professional networking and resources about teaching health policy content, public policy process, and the politics of health policy making in health administration graduate and undergraduate programs, health policy, and public health administration programs. There are 139 members.

Innovative Teaching

With 217 members, the forum works to exchange information and resources in support of facilitating innovative teaching for key competencies and skill sets.

Interprofessional Education

The purpose of the Interprofessional Education (IPE) Forum is to provide a space to encourage and promote practices which advance interprofessional learning experiences as they relate to Healthcare Administration and Healthcare Management. This new Faculty Forum already has 18 members.

Management

The forum's goal is to continually improve research and teaching of core management competencies in the domains of organizational theory and organizational behavior, human resources, strategic thinking, marketing, and creative leadership. The forum has 136 members.

Medical Group Practice/Ambulatory Care

The forum is a resource for teachers, program directors, researchers, and managers offering (a) course materials (e.g., syllabi, case studies, ideas for competency development, and new course content); (b) readings organized by the eight domains of the Body of Knowledge for Medical Practice Management of the Medical Group Management Association/American College of Medical Practice Executives; (c) an online forum for discussing current issues and sharing experiences in teaching and practicing medical group management; and (d) an opportunity to critique and add resources to the network. The forum has 46 members.

Online Teaching and Technology

With 173 members, the forum works to encourage and enhance collaboration and disseminate information regarding information technology use in the classroom.

Post-Acute Care

This forum shares teaching resources to enhance the quality of teaching and attract students with outstanding potential and diverse backgrounds to this critical healthcare segment. There are 61 members.

Public Health

This forum's mission is to promote quality teaching of public health principles and core competencies in health administration programs. There are 109 members.

Quality Improvement

This forum was created to stimulate knowledge exchange about the improvement of health and health services among AUPHA members. There are 139 members.

In addition to these formally endorsed faculty forums, AUPHA supports an Open Forum for all AUPHA members, as well as communities and discussion groups that seek to establish sufficient faculty engagement for promotion to Faculty Forum status.

Chart 9. AUPHA Network Total Annual Log-Ins, 2010–2017

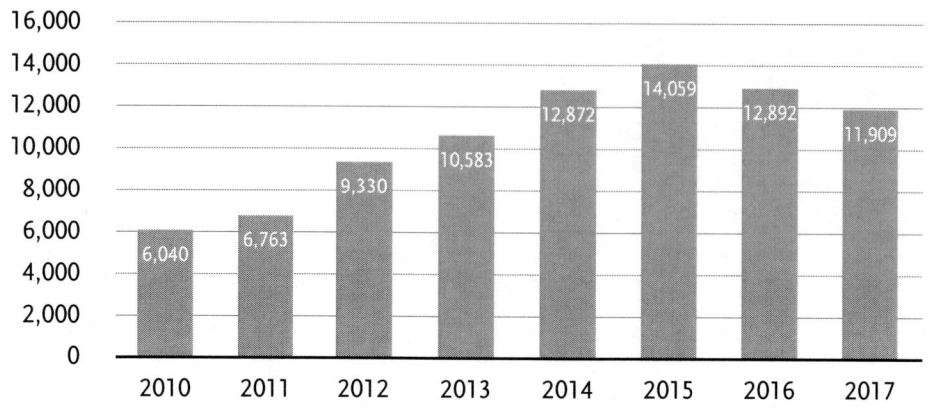

Chart 10. AUPHA Network Total Annual Unique Log-Ins, 2010–2017

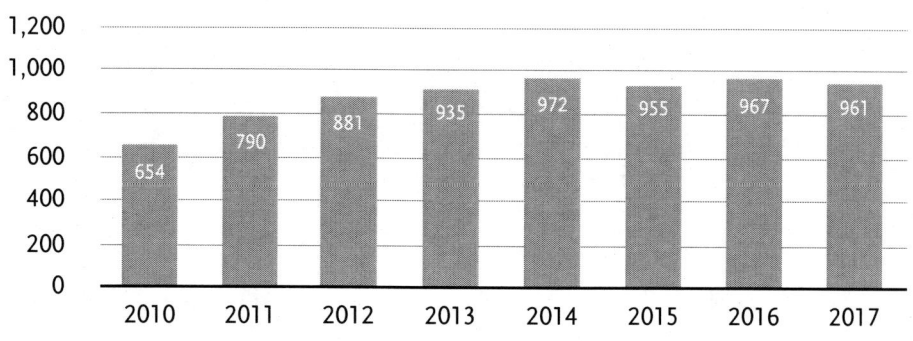

The measurement of engagement for these virtual entities indicates the level of involvement. Chart 10 presents the number of annual log-ins to the AUPHA network, and Chart 11 presents the number of "unique" log-ins. Both are per calendar year, and the data are from 2010 to 2017. The level of activity by these measures is quite high. Nearly 1,000 individual members have engaged with the system during the last four years. Although the number of times they are logging in during the year has declined somewhat, many members are consistently using the system.

Meetings

The second major networking activity that AUPHA supports is our meetings. We host three major events: Annual Meeting, Graduate Program and Practitioner Workshop, and Undergraduate Workshop. The first two meetings occur every year, but the Undergraduate Workshop is held every other year. The location for the Graduate Program and Practitioner Workshop always accompanies the American College of Healthcare Executives (ACHE) Congress on Healthcare Leadership, usually in March in Chicago. The Annual Meeting is in a different location each year, with the intent to rotate geographically so that members do not always travel to the East Coast, West Coast, or Midwest. An Undergraduate program volunteers to host the Undergraduate Workshop; thus, its location varies by the willingness of member programs to host.

- **Annual Meeting.** The Annual Meeting has been a mainstay for AUPHA since its inception. It generates significant interest, and despite rising costs of travel and accommodations, has a large number of registrants each year. The meeting is currently three days long (Wednesday–Friday) and usually occurs in June. It offers significant opportunities for members to present papers in education, think tank, and ignite sessions. It also hosts AUPHA's annual business meeting, the Pattullo Lecture, an awards luncheon, and the William B. Graham Prize address and dinner. Finally, within the program, several groups get a chance to meet, including the Faculty Forums and Upsilon Phi Delta participants. Surrounding the meeting is a partial-day Global Symposium, the on-site AUPHA certification reviews, and a Board meeting prior to the main meeting. Approximately 300 attendees have attended each Annual Meeting for the last several years. See Appendix 5 for a complete list of past Pattullo lecturers.
- **Graduate Program and Practitioner Workshop.** This is a partial-day program that begins with a presentation sponsored jointly by ACHE and AUPHA. The keynote presenter attracts a large number of practitioners attending the Congress and engages the AUPHA academic community.
- **Undergraduate Workshop.** Held every other year, this meeting combines a heavy emphasis on teaching pedagogy and healthcare management content. Over one and a half days, participants share best practices, innovative teaching methods, and new content additions. The program provides significant opportunities to network and build relationships among colleagues from member programs throughout the country. It generally has outside keynote speakers, usually individuals who are practicing healthcare management professionals. They describe how competencies at the undergraduate level become vital in practice.

Certification

AUPHA has engaged in undergraduate certification since the 1990s, and the process has evolved to become an essential form of recognition. Certification assures all external stakeholders that an outside review determined that the program meets or exceeds a set of standards, which assess quality and relevancy. These professionally accepted criteria are set and regularly revised by AUPHA and its members. Certification further attests that the program withstood the rigors of peer review in which experts critically examine curricula, faculty, and educational outcomes. Prospective students look for AUPHA certification when searching for a program to which to commit.

In a process comparable to other specialty program accreditations, programs seeking certification must submit an extensive self-study detailing the program's structure, educational processes, and assessment mechanisms in response to criteria established by AUPHA and the Undergraduate Program Committee. An external peer panel thoroughly examines the applicant program, with the process culminating in a face-to-face meeting at the AUPHA annual conference. The panel's report and recommendations serve as the basis for certifying the program and driving program improvement.

Certification, while similar in process and standards, differs from accreditation in that it does not require a site visit, thus allowing the costs incurred by the program to remain much lower than that of specialty accreditation. Additionally, certification is not required to meet external mandates, allowing AUPHA to remain focused on the unique financial and educational needs of its undergraduate constituents.

The certification process starts with seven eligibility requirements. Eligibility is determined first to eliminate any program not likely to successfully achieve certification. Factors the review committee looks for include where the program is housed, how many faculty it has, and whether the program has graduated any students. Once a program passes the eligibility phase, it is assessed on 28 individual conditions grouped into six major categories:

1. Program structure, faculty, and resources
2. Student support systems
3. Professional and alumni linkages
4. Curriculum and teaching
5. Experiential and applied learning
6. Program evaluation and improvement

See http://www.aupha.org/new-item/certification for a complete list of current certification requirements.

Prizes/Awards
AUPHA offers a number of prizes and awards for students and faculty. Here is a brief description of some of the most notable.

William B. Graham Prize for Health Services Research
Established in 2006, this prize honors the late William B. Graham, longtime CEO of Baxter International. The prize is the highest distinction that researchers in the

health services field can achieve, succeeding the Baxter International Foundation Prize for Health Services Research.

The Graham Prize recognizes an individual's worldwide contributions to improved public health through health services research, particularly research that has a lasting impact on the healthcare system and the way healthcare is delivered. Nominations are actively sought from all parts of the world.

The prize acknowledges the national or international contributions of health services researchers who apply analytic methods to examine and evaluate health services' organization, financing, and/or delivery. The prize focuses on three main areas: health services management, health policy development, and healthcare delivery. A single, major research contribution or a career-long record of achievement may be recognized.

Awarded at AUPHA's Annual Meeting, the Graham Prize consists of an individual award of $25,000 and an additional $25,000 award given to a nonprofit institution designated by the recipient that supports his or her work.

Andrew Pattullo Lecture

Andrew Pattullo, Vice President of the W.K. Kellogg Foundation, was one of the pioneers of the development of professional healthcare management education. After World War II, he and others realized that hospitals suffered from many challenges, including weak management. He subsequently formed commissions through the foundation to study and make recommendations designed to improve the healthcare management education infrastructure. The lecture serves to continue his legacy by enriching the perspectives of educators through the insights of an individual whose views are important to their mission. The lecturer is an individual to whom health administration educators are not otherwise likely to be exposed. The lecture crosses the boundaries of sectors and disciplines, thus bringing insights from outside of the usual focus of the health administration field. This lecture also occurs each year at the beginning of AUPHA's Annual Meeting.

Gary L. Filerman Prize for Educational Leadership

This prize honors Gary L. Filerman, PhD, the first president of AUPHA, for his many years of service to the association and the healthcare management education field. The Filerman Prize recognizes individuals from AUPHA-member programs who have made outstanding contributions to the field; exhibited leadership; and enriched their institutions, students, and health administration education through their work.

Dr. Filerman is a widely recognized authority on management systems and competency development for health systems.

John D. Thompson Prize for Young Investigators

AUPHA established this prize to honor John D. Thompson, a professor of health administration education, who set teaching, commitment to learning, collegial relationships, and health services research standards that are without peer. The Thompson Prize recognizes young faculty from AUPHA-member programs based on their contributions to the research literature in the health services field.

HCA (Hospital Corporation of America) Corris Boyd Scholars Award

Established in 2006, this program provides scholarships to two deserving minority students entering full AUPHA-member programs. The award honors the late Corris Boyd, whose vision of building a better way to live and work through leadership and diversity underpinned many of his accomplishments. Before his premature death from leukemia in 2005, Mr. Boyd worked with hospital management companies and group purchasing organizations. He committed his life to diversity and excellence in healthcare and believed that leadership development is crucial to success. He was also devoted to the success of minority- and women-owned business enterprises.

Bachrach Family Scholarship for Excellence in Health Administration

Created in 2003, this scholarship provides a one-year award (currently $5,000) to a second-year student in an accredited AUPHA program. Preference is given to students whose program completion would not likely be possible without such support. AUPHA has managed this scholarship since 2017.

David and Linda Bachrach are committed to supporting young scholars in pursuit of excellence. They have a special commitment to the advancement of women in leadership roles. To this end, they have not only provided the corpus of an endowment, but also engage in career counseling for each scholar as he or she completes his or her education and embarks on and progresses along a chosen career path. Estate gift commitments are in place to enhance the value of the endowment and ensure perpetual support of the scholarship program, with the expectation that prior Bachrach Family Scholars will continue to provide counsel to those who follow them.

David A. Winston Health Policy Scholarship

This scholarship aims to increase the number and quality of individuals trained in healthcare policy at the state and federal levels by providing financial support to deserving health policy students for furthering their education.

David A. Winston played a significant role in shaping American health policy for 20 years. He served as a bridge between the public sector, which he knew well from experience, and the private sector, in which he deeply believed. He moved comfortably and skillfully in either world. His advice and counsel were sought and accepted by leaders in both sectors, and his knowledge and integrity earned him the respect and trust of the healthcare community.

Upsilon Phi Delta (UPD) Honor Society

This group recognizes, prepares, and rewards students who excel in the study of healthcare management and policy. Approved by the AUPHA Board in October 2008, the society enables member programs to provide high-achieving students with national recognition as they pursue employment or further education. It also recognizes member programs that foster high academic standards. Constituents see that member programs have a demonstrated, active interest in student education and career development. The purposes of UPD include the following:

1. To elevate the standards, ideals, competence, and ethics of professionally educated women and men in health administration and leadership
2. To recognize and encourage scholarship in healthcare administration
3. To recognize students who achieve distinction in healthcare administration studies in universities and colleges
4. To provide financial assistance through scholarships to outstanding students pursuing graduate degrees or professional studies in healthcare administration
5. To motivate academic excellence in students studying healthcare administration
6. To recognize, by means of granting honorary memberships, individuals who have made outstanding contributions to the profession. Such recognitions are to be limited to one person per year.

Publications

AUPHA uses a variety of publications to communicate and disseminate research and other vital health management information. Its primary mechanisms include the *Journal of Health Administration Education (JHAE)* and the *AUPHA Exchange*. Both have been in existence for many years and have migrated from print editions to electronic. *JHAE* is available to all program faculty and individual members as a part of their member benefits. More information about the publication can be found in Chapter 8.

The *AUPHA Exchange* provides a communication vehicle for membership about key issues relevant to the association. Features include program news, association news, and healthcare management employment opportunities. Each edition of the *AUPHA Exchange* contains a relatively uniform set of elements, including a blog from the sitting AUPHA Board Chair, a blog from the current AUPHA President, news on Board activities, information regarding upcoming AUPHA meetings, network information, a call for nominations if relevant, a new member welcome, and program news. AUPHA publishes the *Exchange* about nine times per year and electronically distributes it to all AUPHA faculty, sponsors, and select friends and subscribers.

FUTURE DIRECTION

Pinpointing AUPHA's future is challenging, to say the least. Putting predictions in print suggests foolhardiness; however, recent Board actions hint at a possible direction. In 2015/2016, because of the complexity of issues that AUPHA—and its constituents—continuously face, the Board recognized the need for a more effective structure and a way to better leverage Board member expertise. It initially identified six categories of strategic direction for the association, listed as follows, and developed committees to look into each strategy. These committees have changed since the completion of the strategic plan, but they remain key indicators of the overall direction of AUPHA. The future of AUPHA relies heavily on its past.

- Member Value: Concentrate all activity on providing measurable value to members.
- Graduate Program: Focuses directly on those issues vital to the graduate program membership.
- Undergraduate Program: Focuses directly on those issues relevant to undergraduate program members and in particular on program certification.
- Collaborative Partnership: Develop and strengthen the already strong relationships and collaborative alliances with key organizations throughout the industry.
- Global Leadership: Strengthen our historical linkages with associations representing health management and health management education throughout the globe (see Chapter 7).
- Diversity with Inclusion: Expand efforts to correct imbalances in healthcare management leadership and healthcare management education (see Chapter 5).

Although the pillars have ebbed and flowed over time, how AUPHA works—and will continue to work—to achieve these strategic goals will actively shape its future. As one often asks in considering the position and future prospects of a company or an association, if AUPHA did not exist, would you create it? The answer is a resounding yes because of the many services provided by AUPHA that benefit individual programs and faculty. These services represent benefits to the common or public good and could not be economically provided individually. More importantly, however, AUPHA provides the collective voice for excellence, innovation, collaboration, diversity, and learning—our values.

This history documents many of the accomplishments and ongoing challenges faced by those who worked tirelessly to build AUPHA, develop quality healthcare management education, improve the quality of healthcare management, and ultimately enhance the health of people throughout the world. Clearly, progress has been substantial, but many hurdles remain. AUPHA today has the infrastructure, resources, and tradition of volunteerism to successfully overcome those hurdles and build upon our history. "AUPHA at 100" should be an interesting book that we all hope to be able to read.

ABOUT THE AUTHOR

Gerald L. Glandon, PhD, is President and CEO of the Association of University Programs in Health Administration. He was professor and chair of the Department of Health Services Administration, University of Alabama at Birmingham, from 2001 to 2013. From 1983 through 2000, he had various faculty and leadership roles in the Department of Health Services Management, Rush University, in Chicago, Illinois. He taught health economics, health policy, and courses on health information technology. In addition to teaching and research, he has extensive experience with health management education globally with programs in Albania, Uzbekistan, Turkmenistan, Kazakhstan, and Saudi Arabia.

Appendix 1

Minutes of December 1948 Meeting

MINUTES OF MEETING

of

ASSOCIATION OF UNIVERSITY PROGRAMS IN HOSPITAL ADMINISTRATION

The organizational meeting of the Association of University
Programs in Hospital Administration was held in New York City Dec.
17, 18, 19, 1948. All meetings were held in the Board Room of the
Roosevelt Hospital. Present were:

> Dr. C. C. Clay, representing Yale
> Dr. L. O. Bradley, representing Toronto
> Miss Eugenia Stuart, representing Toronto
> Dr. Frank Bradley, representing Washington University, St. Louis
> Mr. Jim Hamilton, representing Minnesota
> Mr. Jim Stephan, representing Minnesota
> Dr. Malcolm T. MacEachern, representing Northwestern
> Miss Laura G. Jackson, representing Northwestern
> Miss Marguerite Ducker, representing Northwestern
> Dr. John Gorrell, representing Columbia
> Miss Mary Johnson, representing Columbia
> Dr. A. C. Bachmeyer, representing University of Chicago
> Mr. Ray E. Brown, representing University of Chicago
> Mr. Frank R. Shank, representing University of Chicago
> Mr. Graham Davis, as guest, representing Kellogg Foundation

The group convened at 8:00 on the evening of December 17th.
By prior agreement Dr. Arthur C. Bachmeyer was acting chairman.
Mr. Frank R. Shank was named as acting secretary.

Dr. John Gorrell gave the group a resume of the events leading
up to this meeting. This concerned the discussions held at a
breakfast meeting of several of the administration course representatives in Atlantic City in September 1948 at the annual meeting of the
American Hospital Association. It included also the results of a
questionnaire sent by Dr. Gorrell to the several university courses
and regarding a date for this present meeting and the agenda for
discussion. Dr. Gorrell stated that until a definite decision was
reached by the group as to which particular courses would be invited
into the permanent organization he had thought it wise to invite

ORGANIZATIONAL MEETING

REPRESENTATIVES

CHAIRMAN

HISTORY

only the group present, since this group represented those courses
offering a full program leading to a masters degree.

It was thought that the first order of business should be a
discussion of the need for a permanent organization of course representatives, the purpose of such an organization, and other matters
relating to a name, number of meetings, etc. This discussion **PURPOSE OF THIS ORGANIZATION**
brought out the fact that there was a need for regular meetings of
those concerned with the several courses so as to provide an
opportunity for group discussion of common problems, setting of
standards, accreditation, promote development of education in
hospital administration leading to a degree, and the development and
promotion of research in hospital administration.

Dr. Frank Bradley moved that we organize formally and that Mr. **FORMAL ORGANIZATION**
Ray E. Brown, Chairman, Dr. Clem Clay and Dr. John Gorrell be a
committee of three to draw up by-laws for this organization.

It was the opinion of the group that the membership of the
organization should be composed of only those courses conducted by **MEMBERSHIP**
universities and leading to a masters or equivalent degree. These
courses should consist of one academic year in residence and one
calendar year of administrative residency or its equivalent. A
further criteria would be that the major emphasis of member courses
be on the hospital administrators and that this be demonstrated
through a minimum of not less than one-third of the program being
devoted to hospital administration.

It was agreed that there be one annual meeting and such other

meetings as might be required. The group is to be circularized
as to the exact date of each meeting. The most acceptable times seemed
to be December and Spring. Northwestern and University of Chicago
were asked to act as hosts at the meeting to be held in the spring
of 1949 in Chicago.

NUMBER OF
MEETINGS

The group decided that the name "The Association of University
Programs in Hospital Administration" should be adopted since it
most adequately covered the purposes and proposed membership of the
group.

NAME
OF THIS
ORGANIZATION

In order to avoid confusion in the placement of students in
residencies it was agreed that the Course Directors would not make
definite recommendations before February 1 of each year to preceptors
on students finishing in May or June.

RECOMMENDATIONS
TO PRECEPTORS

In order to prevent duplication in the acceptance of students
and permit the students to make their decisions by a certain date,
the courses agreed to make the first notification between April 1
and April 15 on completed applications and the applicant must reply
by May 1. This would also give the courses time to replace cancel-
lations. On May 1 each course will notify all of the other courses
of the names of the students that have been accepted.

NOTIFICATION
OF STUDENT

NOTIFICATION
OF COURSES

The acting secretary was instructed to send notices to all
hospital magazines that the date of April 1 to 15 will be the date
of acceptances of students in hospital administration by courses com-
prising this Association.

NOTIFY
MAGAZINES

Since there is such a wide variance in the number of students in the respective courses some discussion was had as to what the **NUMBER OF STUDENTS** optimum number of students would be. It was finally determined that the factors involved in the determination of the number of students for a particular course were so numerous and complicated that it was agreed that it must be left up to each course to select the optimum number of students for that particular course. At the present time the courses have the following number of students: Yale: 6, Minnesota: 27, Columbia: 26, Chicago: 12, Northwestern: 35, Toronto: 11, Washington University: 13, and California: 8.

Some discussion was had as to what should be the status of a student who served a combined residency and work experience but no **COMBINED RESIDENCY** definite conclusions were reached. Columbia stated that a paid job **AND WORK EXPERIENCE** will decelerate the residency credit for one of their students one-half. In other words, two years in a paid job would be equal to one year of residency. Program adjustments should be necessary for students who serve a residency in specialized hospitals. It is preferable, however, to have the student serve a residency in a general hospital, but it might be to the student's advantage to serve a portion of a year in a specialized hospital.

Some discussion was had as to what the administrative intern should be called. Some courses have called them interns and some **INTERN CHANGED TO** have called them residents. It was the opinion of some that the **RESIDENT** title of administrative resident would be the better and would carry more prestige. It was agreed that all courses should use the same title, and after this discussion the group voted that the name of the administrative <u>intern</u> should be changed to administrative <u>resident</u>.

The question was asked if the preceptor, the hospital, or both should be considered when placing the administrative resident. After some discussion it was agreed that the preceptor in his hospital should be approved and not the preceptor or the hospital alone for taking administrative residents. Some discussion was had as to how many residents should a preceptor be permitted to take. No conclusion was drawn as to the maximum number of residents the preceptor should take. No definite rule could be established because of the variables in each preceptor and his hospital. Among other criteria discussed the following were mentioned as being essential in judging the preceptor: educational attitude, aptitude, philosophy, preferably a fellow, member, or nominee in the American College of Hospital Administrators, and interest and leadership in the hospital field. The preceptor should be advised that to take an administrative resident should be an educational experience.

PRECEPTOR IN HOSPITAL APPROVED

Some discussion was had as to what each course was doing in regard to residency reporting and evaluating. Northwestern University now has informal reporting and evaluating but is working on a form. Columbia requires formal reports from students and also the preceptor. A representative from the Columbia course visits the student in his residency. Yale has informal reports from the students, and also visits the student in his residency. The rest of the courses do not require written reports from the students in residency, but expect an occasional informative letter.

RESIDENCY REPORTING AND EVALUATING

Discussion was had as to what was being done as to testing applicants for the courses. The types of testing devices were discussed, and the following types are used by Columbia: Kuder Preference Record (Vocational), Kuder Preference Record (Personal), Cordall: Test of Practical Judgment, Minnesota T-S-E, Wonderlic Personnel Test -- Form E (time limit), Adams and Lepley: The Personal Audit.

TESTING
DEVICES

All of the above tests except Wonderlic are obtained from Science Research Association, 228 S. Wabash Avenue, Chicago 4, Illinois. The Wonderlic test is obtained from E. F. Wonderlic, 750 Grove Street, Glencoe, Illinois. Miss Mary Johnson states that she does not believe the Wonderlic is worth the effort, but they are using it primarily to check with the Cornell School of Hotel Administration. Miss Johnson advised that she would circularize a copy of these tests.

Discussion was had as to the requirements for admission for students. Northwestern University requires the following courses before completing the Hospital Administration course: Economics, Sociology, Finance, Psychology, Biology, Statistics. Columbia requires a B. A. or equivalent. Yale requires some biological and physical science, and a reading knowledge of French or German. In addition the students are required to take a graduate record examination. Toronto, Washington, University of Chicago, and Minnesota require a B. A. or equivalent and accounting is almost a requisite.

REQUIREMENTS
FOR ADMISSION

Dr. Clem Clay asked if a general statement of prerequisites

could be made so that each course could agree when writing to the
students. No recommendations of specific requirements were made   PREREQUISITES
and it was the general opinion that the broader the program the
better, but all agreed that essentially the general requirements
of each school would govern.

Some discussion was had as to what part grades should play in
the selection of a student. It was agreed that grades per se were   GRADES
not sufficient criteria but that personality, character and grades
should all be considered in selecting the student. Previous work
experience in hospitals should also be given serious consideration,   EXPERIENCE
as well as general work experience, but particularly work experience
in hospitals. The age should be preferably 25 to 35 years, but   AGE
it was recognized that maturity cannot always be judged by years
alone   None of the courses bar women but all would limit to one
or two in each class, due mainly to the difficulty in placing women   SEX
in the field of hospital administration. Several courses have taken
Negroes, but in most cases these have jobs to go back to. Foreign   RACE
names have been found to be a handicap to placing students.   FOREIGN
NAMES

At the request of Dr. John Gorrell and Dr. Clem Clay, Miss
Grace White, Professor of Medical Social Work, New York School of
Social Work, Columbia University, New York City, and Miss Elizabeth   REPORT
ON
Rice, formerly Director of Social Service, Grace New Haven Community   MEDICAL
SOCIAL
Hospital, New Haven, Connecticut, presented a tentative report of the   SERVICE
Subcommittee of the American Association of Medical Social Workers on
the Teaching of Students in Hospital Administration.

The meeting adjourned Sunday afternoon, December 19 to reconvene ADJOURNMENT
in Chicago in the spring.

Appendix 2

AUPHA Chairs

Years	Name	Organization
1948–1949	Arthur C. Bachmeyer, MD	University of Chicago
1949–1950	Malcolm T. MacEachern, MD	Northwestern University
1950–1951	John Gorell, MD	Columbia University
1951–1953	James A. Hamilton	University of Minnesota
1953–1954	G. Harvey Agnew, MD	University of Toronto
1954–1955	Frank R. Bradley, MD	Washington University
1955–1956	George S. Buis	Yale University
1956–1957	John S. Flanagan, SJ	Saint Louis University
1957–1958	Richard J. Stull	University of California, Berkeley
1958–1959	John R. McGibony, MD	University of Pittsburgh
1959–1960	Robert Hudgens	Medical College of Virginia/Virginia Commonwealth University
1960–1961	Colonel Glenn K. Smith	U.S. Army/Baylor University
1961–1962	Gerhard Hartman, PhD	University of Iowa
1962–1963	Thomas B. Fitzpatrick	University of Michigan
1963–1964	Gerald LaSalle, MD	University of Montreal
1964–1965	Frederick H. Gibbs, MSc	The George Washington University
1965–1966	George Bugbee	University of Chicago
1966–1967	Ray E. Brown, MBA	Duke University
1967–1968	Lawrence A. Hill, MHA	University of Michigan
1968–1969	John D. Thompson, RN, MS	Yale University
1969–1970	F. Burns Roth, MD	University of Toronto
1970–1971	Paul R. Donnelly	Saint Louis University
1971–1972	Bright M. Dornblaser, MHA	University of Minnesota
1972–1973	David B. Starkweather, DrPH	University of California, Berkeley
1973–1974	James O. Hepner, PhD	Washington University
1974–1975	John R. Griffith, MBA	University of Michigan
1975–1976	Walter M. Burnett, PhD	Tulane University
1976–1977	B. Jon Jaeger, PhD	Duke University
1977–1978	Stuart A. Wesbury, PhD	University of Missouri–Columbia
1978–1979	Lawrence D. Prybil, PhD	Medical College of Virginia/Virginia Commonwealth University
1979–1980	William L. Dowling, PhD	University of Washington–Seattle
1980–1981	Samuel Levey, PhD	University of Iowa
1981–1982	Stephen F. Loebs, PhD	The Ohio State University

Years	Name	Organization
1982–1983	R. Hopkins Holmberg, PhD	Boston University
1983–1984	Thomas C. Dolan, PhD	Saint Louis University
1984–1985	Lee F. Seidel, PhD	University of New Hampshire
1985–1986	Barry R. Greene, PhD	University of Florida
1986–1987	Gordon D. Brown, PhD	University of Missouri–Columbia
1987–1988	Peggy Leatt, PhD	University of Toronto
1988–1989	Charles J. Austin, PhD	University of Alabama at Birmingham
1989–1990	James D. Suver, DBA	University of Colorado Denver
1990–1991	Richard S. Kurz, PhD	Saint Louis University
1991–1992	Mary E. Stefl, PhD	Trinity University
1992–1993	Deborah A. Freund, PhD	Indiana University
1993–1994	John W. Seavey, PhD	University of New Hampshire
1994–1995	Eugene S. Schneller, PhD	Arizona State University
1995–1996	Cynthia Carter Haddock, PhD	University of Kansas
1996–1997	Mary Richardson, PhD	University of Washington
1997–1998	John R.C. Wheeler, PhD	University of Michigan
1998–1999	Janet Reagan, PhD	California State University, Northridge
1999–2000	Ray Davis, PhD	University of Kansas
2000–2002	David J. Fine, MHA, FACHE	University of Alabama at Birmingham
2002–2004	G. Ross Baker, PhD	University of Toronto
2004–2005	Diana W. Hilberman, DrPH	University of California, Los Angeles
2005–2006	Leonard Friedman, PhD	Oregon State University
2006–2007	Dean G. Smith, PhD	University of Michigan
2007–2008	Sharon Buchbinder, RN, PhD	Towson University
2008–2009	John Lowe, PhD	Simmons College
2009–2010	Grant Savage, PhD	University of Missouri
2011–2012	Peter Fitzpatrick, PhD	Clayton State University
2012–2013	Sharon Schweikhart, PhD	The Ohio State University
2013–2014	Ken Johnson, PhD	Weber State University
2014–2015	Tom Vaughn, PhD	University of Iowa
2015–2016	Christy Harris Lemak, PhD	University of Alabama at Birmingham
2016–2017	Diane M. Howard, PhD	Rush University
2017–2018	Keith J. Benson, PhD	Winthrop University

Appendix 3

AUPHA Presidents

Years	Name
1965–1993	Gary L. Filerman
1994–1997	Henry Fernandez
1998–1999	Janet E. Porter
2000–2003	Jeptha W. Dalston
2004–2012	Lydia Middleton (Reed)
2013–present	Gerald L. Glandon

Appendix 4

William B. Graham Prize for Health Services Research Recipients

Year	Winner	Organization
1986	Avedis Donabedian, MD, MPH	University of Michigan
1987	Brian Abel-Smith, PhD	University of London
1988	Robert Brook, MD, ScD	Rand Corporation/University of California, Los Angeles
	Joseph P. Newhouse, PhD	Rand Corporation/University of California, Los Angeles
1989	Mickey Eisenberg, MD, PhD	University of Washington
1990	Rosemary Stevens, PhD	University of Pennsylvania
1991	Victor R. Fuchs, PhD	Stanford University
1992	John D. Thompson, RN, MS	Yale University
	Robert B. Fetter, DBA	Yale University
1993	John Wennberg, MD, MPH	Dartmouth College
1994	Alain C. Enthoven, PhD	Stanford University
1995	Stephen M. Shortell, PhD	University of California, Berkeley
1996	Kerr L. White, MD	University of Virginia
1997	David Mechanic, PhD	Rutgers University
1998	Harold S. Luft, PhD	University of California, San Francisco
1999	Ronald Andersen, PhD	University of California, Los Angeles
	Odin Anderson, PhD	University of Wisconsin–Madison
2000	Karen Davis, PhD	The Commonwealth Fund
2001	Robert G. Evans, PhD	University of British Columbia
2002	John M. Eisenberg, MD, MBA	Agency for Healthcare Research and Quality
2003	Robert J. Blendon, ScD	Harvard University
2004	Barbara Starfield, MD, MPH	Johns Hopkins University
2005	David L. Sackett, OC, MD, FRSC, FRCP	Trout Research Institute
2006	Linda H. Aiken, PhD, FAAN, FRCN, RN	University of Pennsylvania
2007	Donald M. Berwick, MD, MPP	Institute for Healthcare Improvement
2008	Sir Michael G. Marmot, MBBS, MPH, PhD	University College London
2009	Carolyn M. Clancy, MD	Agency for Healthcare Research and Quality
2010	Uwe E. Reinhardt, PhD	Princeton University
2011	Edward H. Wagner, MD	Group Health Research Institute
2012	Mark V. Pauly, PhD	University of Pennsylvania
2013	Dorothy P. Rice, ScD	University of California, San Francisco

Year	Winner	Organization
2014	Stuart H. Altman, PhD	Brandeis University
2015	Anthony J. Culyer, CBE, BA, Hon DEcon, Hon FRCP, FRSA, FMedSci	University of York
	Alan Maynard, OBE, BPhil, Hon DSc, Hon LLD, Hon MFPHM, MMEDSci	University of York
2016	John K. Iglehart	*Health Affairs*
2017	David Blumenthal, MD	The Commonwealth Fund

Note: Until 2007, this award was the Baxter Health Services Research Prize.

Appendix 5

Pattullo Lecturers

Year	Name	Title	Organization
1983	Harlan Cleveland, PhD	Professor	University of Minnesota
1984	Stuart H. Altman, PhD	Dean	Brandeis University
1985	Bruce C. Vladeck, PhD	President	United Hospital Fund of New York
1986	Steven Muller, PhD	President	Johns Hopkins University
1987	The Honourable Marc Lalonde, PC, OC, QC	Former Minister of Health and Welfare	Government of Canada
1988	Robert G. Petersdorf, MD	President	Association of American Medical Colleges
1989	Norman A. Brown, PhD	President and Chief Programming Officer	W.K. Kellogg Foundation
1990	Arnold S. Relman, MD	Editor	*New England Journal of Medicine*
1991	William C. Richardson, PhD	President	Johns Hopkins University
1992	Margaret E. Mahoney	President	The Commonwealth Fund
1993	William L. Roper, MD, MPH	Director	Centers for Disease Control and Prevention
1994	Robert Evans, PhD	Professor	University of British Columbia
1995	Walter J. McNerney, MHA	Professor	Northwestern University
1996	Robert Sigmond, BA, MA	Advisor on Hospital Affairs	Blue Cross and Blue Shield Association
1997	Sandra Hernandez, MD	Professor	University of Michigan
1998	John R. Griffith, MBA, FACHE	Professor	University of Michigan
1999	Jo Ivey Boufford, MD	Dean	Robert F. Wagner Graduate School of Public Service, New York University
2000	Gail Warden, MHA	CEO	Henry Ford Health System
2001	Ross Baker, PhD	Professor	University of Toronto
	John Eisenberg, MD, MBA	Director	Agency for Health Care Policy and Research
	Harry Hertz, BS, PhD	Director Emeritus	Baldrige National Quality Program
	John King, FACHE	Advisor	Legacy Health Systems
	Mary Jean Ryan	CEO	SSM Health Care
	Horst Schultze, PhD	President	Ritz Carlton Hotel Company

Year	Name	Title	Organization
2002	William Dwyer, MBA	Divisional Vice President	Abbott Health Systems Division, Abbott Laboratories
2003	The Honourable Marc Lalonde, PC, OC, QC	Former Minister of Health and Welfare	Government of Canada
2004	Steven Muller, PhD	President	Johns Hopkins University
2005	Risa Lavizzo-Mourey, MD	President and CEO	Robert Wood Johnson Foundation
2006	Kenneth H. Cohn, MD, MBA, FACS	Associate Professor of Surgery and Chief of Surgical Oncology	VA Hospital at White River Junction
2007	Ronald A. Berk, PhD	Professor of Biostatistics and Measurement	Johns Hopkins University
2008	Karen Davis, PhD	President	The Commonwealth Fund
2009	Regina E. Herzlinger, PhD	Nancy R. McPherson Professor of Business Administration	Harvard Business School
2010	George C. Halvorson, PhD	Chairman and CEO	Kaiser Foundation Health Plan, Inc.
2011	Uwe E. Reinhardt, PhD	James Madison Professor of Political Economy	Princeton University
2012	Ann Bancroft	Polar Explorer and Founder	Ann Bancroft Foundation
2013	Carrie Owen Plietz, MHA	CEO	Sutter Medical Center Sacramento
2014	Major General David Rubenstein, MHA, FACHE	Major General (retired) and Clinical Associate Professor	Texas State University
2015	Herminia Palacio, MD	Director of Leadership and Human Capital	Robert Wood Johnson Foundation
2016	Kevin L. Alexander, OD, PhD, FAAO	President	Marshall B. Ketchum University
2017	Josh Luke, PhD, FACHE	Chief Strategy Officer	Nelson Hardiman Healthcare Law

Appendix 6

John D. Thompson Prize for Young Investigators Recipients

Year	Winner	Organization
1991	Michael A. Morrisey, PhD	University of Alabama at Birmingham
1992	Thomas H. Rice, PhD	University of California, Los Angeles
1993	David Dranove, PhD	Northwestern University
1994	No awardee	
1995	Peter C. Coyte, PhD	University of Toronto
1996	Jacqueline S. Zinn, PhD	Temple University
1997	No awardee	
1998	Michael Chernew, PhD	University of Michigan
1999	Richard A. Hirth, PhD	University of Michigan
2000	Brian Weiner, PhD	University of North Carolina at Chapel Hill
2001	William Dow, PhD	University of North Carolina at Chapel Hill
2002	Shoou-Yih Daniel Lee, PhD Dennis P. Scanlon, PhD	University of North Carolina at Chapel Hill The Pennsylvania State University
2003	Elizabeth Bradley, PhD	Yale School of Medicine
2004	David C. Grabowski, PhD	University of Alabama at Birmingham
2005	John Cawley, PhD	Cornell University
2006	Kevin Volpp, MD, PhD	University of Pennsylvania
2007	Kosali Ilayperuma Simon, PhD	Cornell University
2008	Michael Davern, PhD Rachel M. Werner, MD, PhD	University of Minnesota University of Pennsylvania
2010	Daniel Eisenberg, PhD Jonathan Ketcham, PhD	University of Michigan Arizona State University
2011	Hector Rodriguez, PhD	University of California, Los Angeles
2012	George L. Wehby, PhD	University of Iowa
2013	Diana M. Bowman, LLB, PhD	University of Michigan
2014	Holly Jarman, PhD	University of Michigan
2015	Larry Hearld, PhD	University of Alabama at Birmingham
2016	Brad Wright, PhD	University of Iowa
2017	David K. Jones, PhD	Boston University

Appendix 7

Corris Boyd Scholars

Year	Winner	Organization
2006	Marcus Smith Jennifer R. Bonds	Cornell University University of North Carolina at Chapel Hill
2007	Andrea N. Gwyn Kenneth M. West II	Virginia Commonwealth University Georgetown University
2008	Essein Ukanna Shruti D. Kothari	University of Michigan University of California, Berkeley
2009	Lawrence Smith Nupur Agrawal	Cornell University Columbia University
2010	Jonathan Liu William English	Columbia University University of Alabama at Birmingham
2011	Prince Baawuah Jared Dunlap	University of Michigan Columbia University
2012	Carolina Garcia Mohamed Jalloh	Northwestern University University of North Carolina at Chapel Hill
2013	Carolina de la Puente Crystal Sanford	The George Washington University University of Southern California
2014	Shekinah Bell Jennifer N. Dingle	University of Michigan University of Michigan
2015	Gloria Coicou Jacqueline Gallardo	Cornell University University of Southern California
2016	Lee Salazar Patara Williams	University of Washington–Seattle Xavier University
2017	Cameron Gabriel Taylor Jordan Onyeka Okeke	University of Minnesota Columbia University Johns Hopkins University

Appendix 8

Gary L. Filerman Prize for Educational Leadership Recipients

Year	Winner	Organization
1996	James D. Suver, DBA	University of Colorado–Denver
1997	Peggy Leatt, PhD	University of North Carolina at Chapel Hill
1998	Gordon D. Brown, PhD	University of Missouri–Columbia
1999	Anthony R. Kovner, PhD	New York University
2000	Stephen F. Loebs, PhD	The Ohio State University
2001	Vernon Weckwerth, PhD	University of Minnesota
2002	John R. Griffith, MBA, FACHE	University of Michigan
2003	Charles J. Austin, PhD	University of Alabama at Birmingham
2004	Mary E. Stefl, PhD	Trinity University
2005	Thomas G. Rundall, PhD	University of California, Berkeley
2006	S. Robert Hernandez, DrPH	University of Alabama at Birmingham
2007	G. Ross Baker, PhD	University of Toronto
2008	James W. Begun, PhD	University of Minnesota
2009	Douglas Conrad, PhD	University of Washington–Seattle
2010	Eugene S. Schneller, PhD	Arizona State University
2011	Barry R. Greene, PhD	University of Iowa
2012	John R. C. Wheeler, PhD	University of Michigan
2013	Stephen Mick, PhD	Virginia Commonwealth University
2014	Janet Reagan, PhD	California State University, Northridge
2015	Richard Lichtenstein, PhD	University of Michigan
2016	Peter Butler, MHSA	Rush University
2017	Sherril B. Gelmon, DrPH	Oregon Health Sciences University and Portland State University

Appendix 9

Special Issues of the *Journal of Health Administration Education*

Issue	Volume/ Number	Title	Guest Editors
Winter 1987	Vol. 5, No. 1	Management of Population Planning Programs	Sagar Jain, PhD, and Michael Markowitz
Summer 1987	Vol. 5, No. 3	Multi-Institutional Systems Management	Jeffrey Alexander, PhD
Summer 1988	Vol. 6, No. 3	NHS Management: Beyond the Griffiths Report to Current Issues	David Thomson, PhD
Summer 1989	Vol. 7, No. 3	Teaching and Using Research Methods in Health Administration	Arnold D. Kauzny, PhD
Winter 1990	Vol. 8, No. 1	Information Systems Education for Future Health Services Administrators	Charles J. Austin, PhD, and Brian T. Malec, PhD
Spring 1990	Vol. 8, No. 2	Undergraduate Education in Health Administration	Janet Thompson
Fall 1990	Vol. 8, No. 4	Strategic Alignment of Health Care Organizations: Management Case Studies	Douglas A. Conrad, PhD, and Geoffrey A. Hoarre, PhD
Spring 1991	Vol. 9, No. 2	Health Administration in Australia	Colin Grant and Helen Lapsey
Winter 1992	Vol. 10, No. 1	Aids: The Management Challenge for the 21st Century	Sherril B. Gelmon, DrPH
Fall 1992	Vol. 10, No. 4	Long-Term Care Administration: New Views for the Future	Richard M. Shewchuk, PhD, and Nancy E. Hinkley, EdD
Spring 1993	Vol. 11, No. 2	Postgraduate Management Development	Lawrence D. Prybil and Gail L. Warden
Summer 1994	Vol. 12, No. 3	Community Benefit Programs for Health Care Organizations	Anthony Kovner, PhD
Fall 1994	Vol. 12, No. 4	Health Sector Management Capacity Building in Central and Eastern Europe	James A. Rice, PhD
Winter 1995	Vol. 13, No. 1	Quality Improvement in Health Management Education	Bright Dornblaster, MHA, and Joel Shalowitz, MD
Fall 1995	Vol. 13, No. 4	Accreditation in the Nineties, Part 1	Peggy Leatt, PhD, and Barry R. Greene, PhD
Winter 1996	Vol. 14, No. 1	Accreditation in the Nineties, Part 2	Peggy Leatt, PhD, and Barry R. Greene, PhD

Issue	Volume/Number	Title	Guest Editors
Spring 1996	Vol. 14, No. 2	Provider Payment Reforms in Russia: The Economic Lever for Health Sector Performance Improvement	James A. Rice, PhD, with Courtney S. Roberts, MA
Summer 1997	Vol. 15, No. 3	Health Management Education and Development: Partnership in Central and Eastern Europe, Part 1	William E. Aaronson, PhD, and Daniel J. West Jr., PhD, FACHE
Spring 1998	Vol. 16, No. 2	Health Management Education and Development: Partnership in Central and Eastern Europe, Part 2	William E. Aaronson, PhD, and Daniel J. West Jr., PhD, FACHE
Winter 2001	Vol. 19, No. 1	The State of Online Education in Health Administration Programs	Philip S. DiSalvio, EdD, and Farrokh Alemi, PhD
Summer 2001	Vol. 19, No. 3	The State of Doctoral Education in Health Administration and Policy	Myron D. Fottler, PhD, and James A. Johnson, PhD
Fall 2003	Vol. 20, No. 4	Teaching Evidence-Based Healthcare Management	Anthony R. Kovner, PhD
Summer 2007	Vol. 24, No. 3	The State of Doctoral Education in Health Administration and Policy Revisited	Myron Fottler, PhD, and Joel Lee, DrPH
Fall 2014	Vol. 31, No. 4	Postgraduate Healthcare Management Fellowships	Diane M. Howard, PhD, and Ana Maria Lomperis, PhD
Spring 2015	Vol. 32, No. 2	Essays in Honor of Stephen S. Mick, PhD, FACHE	Dean G. Smith, PhD, and Mark L. Diana, PhD
Fall 2015	Vol. 32, No. 4	Online Healthcare Management Education	Linda J. Mast, PhD, Anne Hewitt, PhD, Stephen Gambescia, PhD, and Donald L. Zimmerman, PhD
Spring 2017	Vol. 34, No. 2	Diversity and Inclusion, Part 1	Keith Elder, PhD, and Laurie Shanderson, PhD
Summer 2017	Vol. 34, No. 3	Diversity and Inclusion, Part 2	Keith Elder, PhD, and Laurie Shanderson, PhD

Appendix 10

Graduate Program and Practitioner Workshop Keynote Speakers

Year	Name	Title	Organization
2000	Gary A. Mecklenburg, CHE	President and CEO	Northwestern Memorial Hospital
2001	Panel National Summit		
2002	Gail L. Warden, MHA, FACHE	Chairman and CEO	National Center for Healthcare Leadership
2003	Lawrence D. Prybil, PhD	Professor and Associate Dean	University of Iowa
2004	Lou Rubino, PhD	Professor	California State University, North Ridge
2005	Diana Hilberman, DrPH	Professor	University of California, Los Angeles School of Public Health
2006	Mary E. Stefl, PhD	Professor, Department of Health Management and Policy	Trinity University
2007	Anthony R. Kovner, PhD	Professor Emeritus of Public and Health Management	New York University Robert F. Wagner Graduate School of Public Service
2008	Donald Berwick, MD	President and CEO	Institute for Healthcare Improvement
2009	Larry Mullins, DHA	President and CEO	Samaritan Health Systems
2010	John R. Griffith, MBA	Professor, Department of Health Management and Policy	University of Michigan
2011	Cynthia Hahn, FACHE, CAE	Vice President of Membership	American College of Healthcare Executives
2012	Major General David Rubenstein, FACHE	Commanding General	U.S. Army Medical Department Center & School
2013	John Lynch III, MHA	President and CEO	Main Line Health
2014	Nancy Schlichting, MBA	Chief Executive Officer	Henry Ford Health System
2015	Jessie Tucker III , PhD	Administrator	Lyndon B. Johnson Memorial Hospital
2016	Margaret O'Kane	President	National Committee for Quality Assurance
2017	Halee Fischer-Wright, MD	President and CEO	Medical Group Management Association
2018	David Nash, MD, MBA	Dean	Jefferson College of Population Health

Note: Before 2017, the workshop was called the Leaders Conference.

Appendix 11

AUPHA Board Members, 2002–2017

Name	Organization
Mark Allen, MBA	Boston University
Ross Baker, PhD	**University of Toronto**
James Begun, PhD	University of Minnesota
Keith J. Benson, MHA, PhD	**Winthrop University**
Lavonna Blair-Lewis, PhD	University of Southern California
Nancy Borkowski, DBA	University of Alabama at Birmingham
Diane Brannon, PhD	The Pennsylvania State University
Charles Brecher, PhD	New York University
Sharon Buchbinder, PhD	**Stevenson University**
Claudia Campbell, PhD	Tulane University
Rosemary Caron, PhD	University of New Hampshire
Caryl Carpenter, PhD	Widener University
Leigh Cellucci, PhD	East Carolina University
Dolores Clement, DrPH	Virginia Commonwealth University
Julia Costich, JD, PhD	University of Kentucky
Gina Cronin, MHA	Cleveland Clinic
Simone Cummings, PhD	Webster University
Ray Davis, PhD	**University of Kansas**
Mark Diana, PhD	Tulane University
Rupert Evans, DHA	Governors State University
Tracy Farnsworth, EdD	Idaho State University
David Fine, MHA, FACHE	**University of Alabama at Birmingham**
Peter Fitzpatrick, PhD	**Clayton State University**
Jeffrey Flaks, MHA	Hartford Hospital
Eric Ford, PhD	Johns Hopkins University
Brenda Freshman, PhD	California State University, Long Beach
Leonard Friedman, PhD	**The George Washington University**
Jackie Gaines, MSN	Studer Group
Dan Gentry, PhD	University of Iowa
Raymond Grady, MHA, FACHE	Methodist Hospitals
Kyle Grazier, DrPH	University of Michigan
S. Robert Hernandez, PhD	University of Alabama at Birmingham
Diana Hilberman, DrPH	**University of California, Los Angeles**
Brooke Hollis, MBA	Cornell University

Name	Organization
Diane M. Howard, PhD, MPH	**Rush University**
James Johnson, PhD	Central Michigan University
Ken Johnson, PhD	**Weber State University**
Kerry Kilpatrick, PhD	University of North Carolina at Chapel Hill
Joel Lee, DrPH	University of Georgia
Christy Harris Lemak, PhD	**University of Alabama at Birmingham**
John Lowe, PhD	**Simmons College**
Mary Kay Madsen, PhD	University of Wisconsin–Milwaukee
Brenda Stevenson Marshall, PhD	Cleveland State University
Michael R. Meacham, JD	Medical University of South Carolina
Steve Mick, PhD	Virginia Commonwealth University
Carol Molinari, PhD	University of Baltimore
Craig Nesta, JD, MBA	Brigham and Women's Hospital
Mark Pauly, PhD	University of Pennsylvania
Sandy Potthoff, PhD	University of Minnesota
Bernardo Ramirez, MD	University of Central Florida
Catherine Robbins, MBA, FHFMA	Simmons College
Lou Rubino, PhD	California State University, Northridge
Thomas Rundall, PhD	University of California, Berkeley
Grant Savage, PhD	**University of Alabama at Birmingham**
Sharon Schweikhart, PhD	**The Ohio State University**
Dean Smith, PhD	**University of Michigan**
Mary E. Stefl, PhD	Trinity University
Quint Studer, MS	Studer Group
Andy Sumner, PhD	Georgia State University
Rodney Taylor	Maryland Department of Health and Hygiene
Jon Thompson, PhD	James Madison University
Thomas Vaughn, PhD	**University of Iowa**
Douglas Wakefield, PhD	University of Missouri
Carla Wiggins, PhD	Weber State University
Suzanne Wood, PhD	University of Washington

Note: Boldface indicates a Board chair.

AUPHA Photos

AUPHA CHAIRS

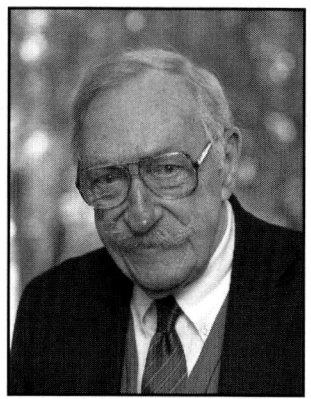

John D. Thompson, RN, MS
1968–1969

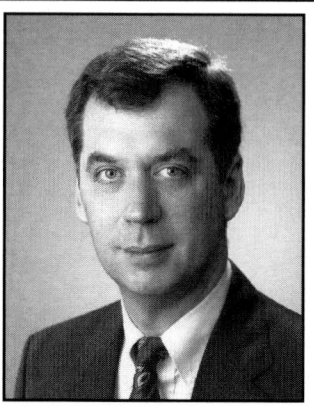

Thomas C. Dolan, PhD
1983–1984

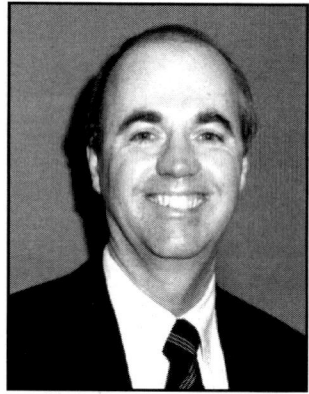

John W. Seavy, PhD
1993–1994

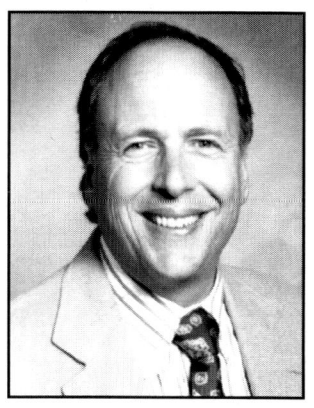

Eugene S. Schneller, PhD
1994–1995

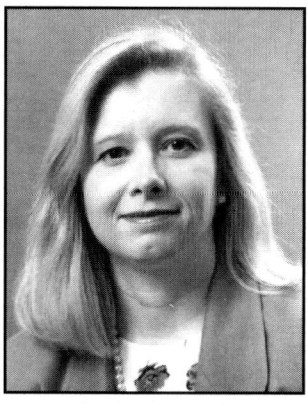

Cynthia Carter Haddock, PhD
1995–1996

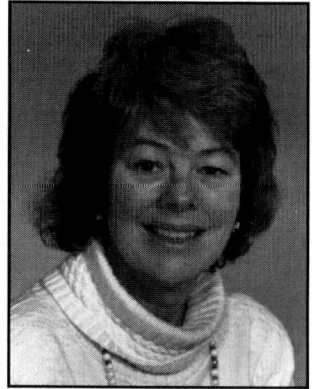

Mary Richardson, PhD
1996–1997

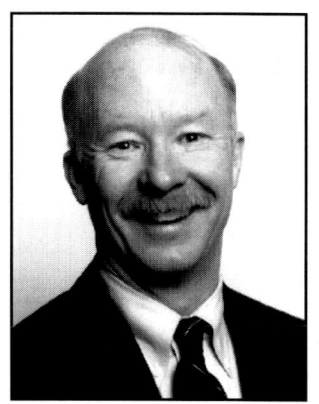

John (Jack) R. C. Wheeler, PhD
1997–1998

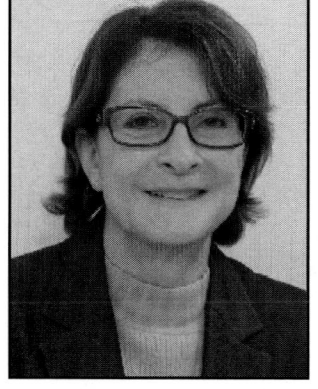

Janet Reagan, PhD
1998–1999

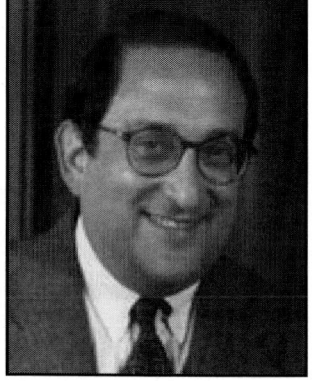

David J. Fine, MHA
2000–2002

AUPHA CHAIRS *(continued)*

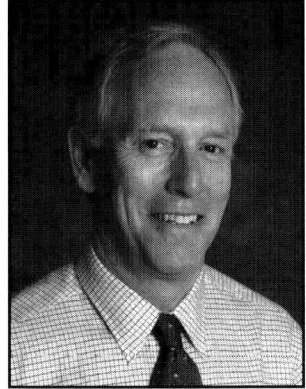

G. Ross Baker, PhD
2002–2003

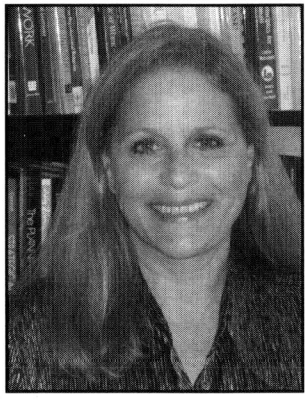

Diana W. Hilberman, PhD
2004–2005

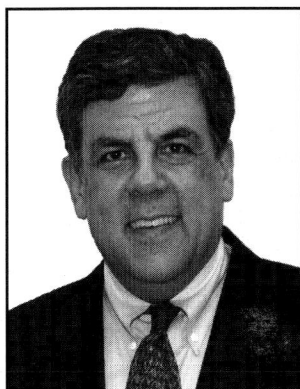

Leonard Friedman, PhD
2005–2006

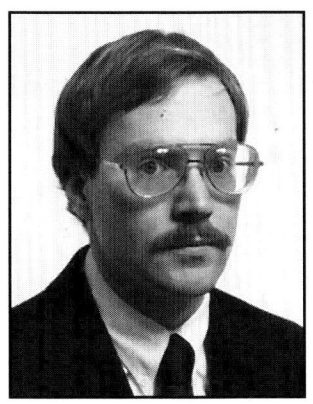

Dean G. Smith, PhD
2006–2007

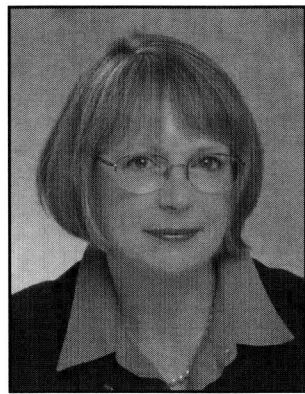

Sharon Buchbinder, RN, PhD
2007–2008

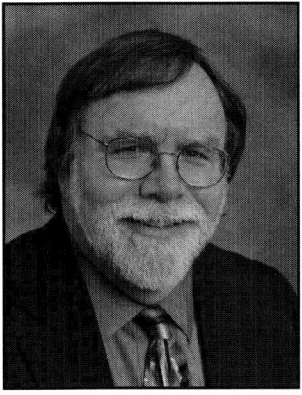

John Lowe, PhD
2008–2009

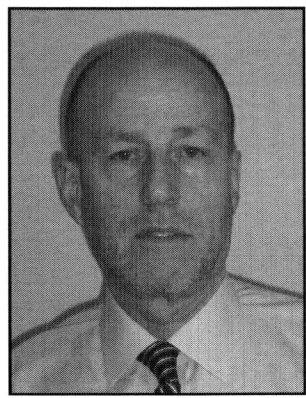

Peter Fitzpatrick, PhD
2011–2012

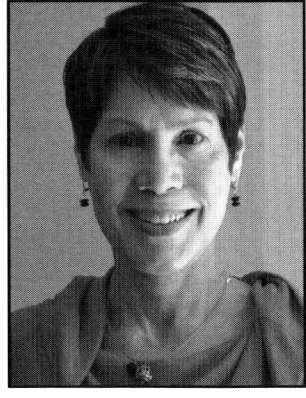

Sharon Schweikhart, PhD
2012–2013

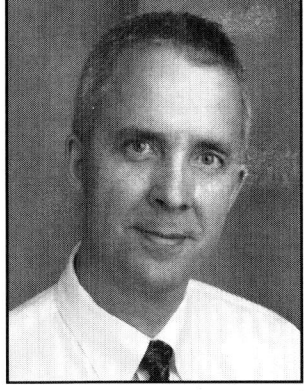

Kenneth W. Johnson, PhD
2013–2014

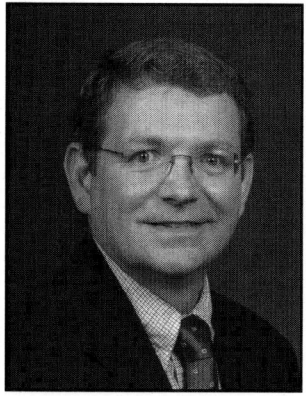

Thomas Vaughn, PhD
2014–2015

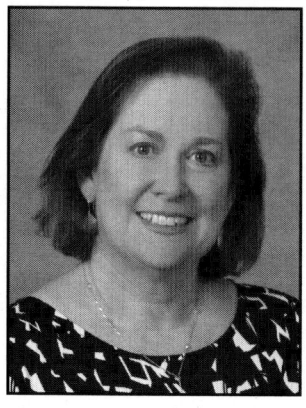

Christy Harris Lemak, PhD
2015–2016

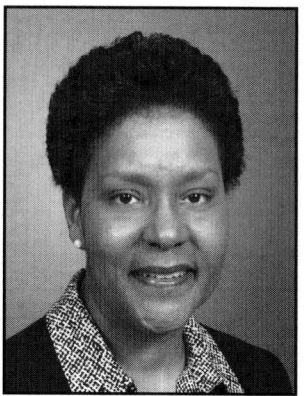

Diane M. Howard, PhD
2016–2017

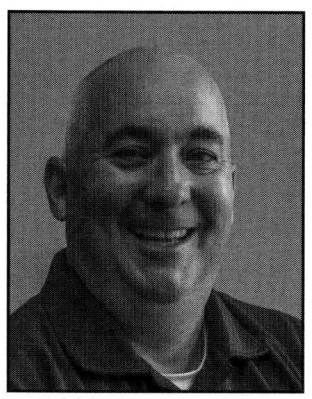

Keith J. Benson, PhD
2017–2018

AUPHA PRESIDENTS

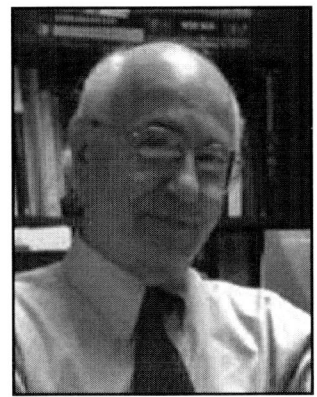

Gary L. Filerman, PhD
1965–1993

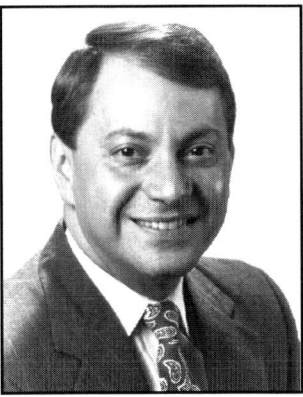

Henry Fernandez, PhD
1994–1997

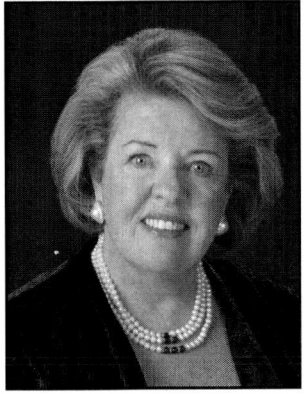

Janet E. Porter, PhD
1998–1999

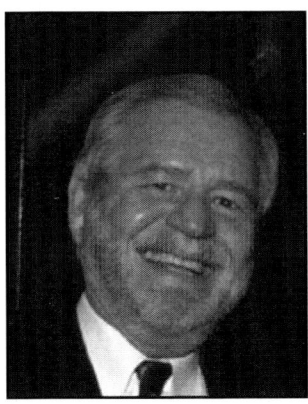

Jeptha W. Dalston, PhD
2000–2003

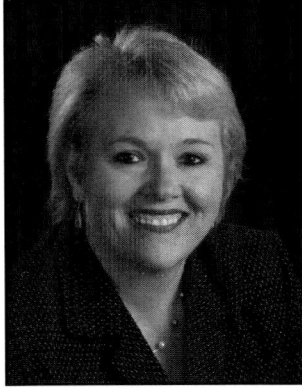

Lydia Middleton (Reed),
CAE, MBA
2004–2012

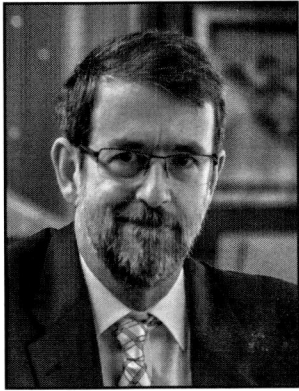

Gerald L. Glandon, PhD
2013–present

AUPHA 60TH ANNIVERSARY AT THE 2008 ANNUAL MEETING IN CHICAGO

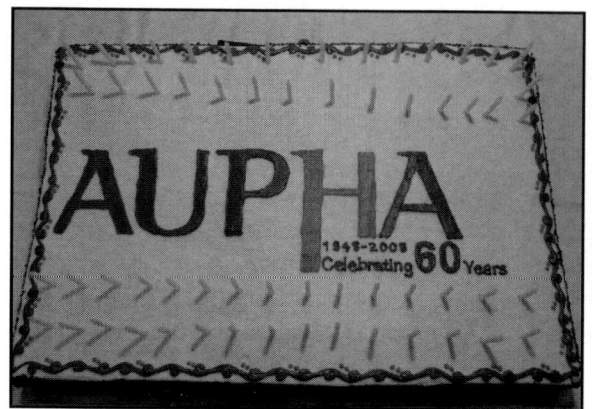

60th anniversary cake

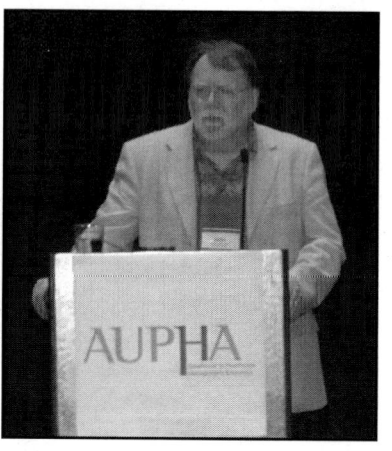

2008 Board Chair John Lowe, PhD

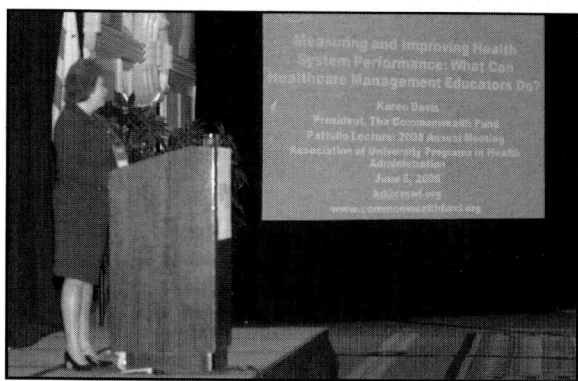

2008 Pattullo Lecturer Karen Davis, PhD

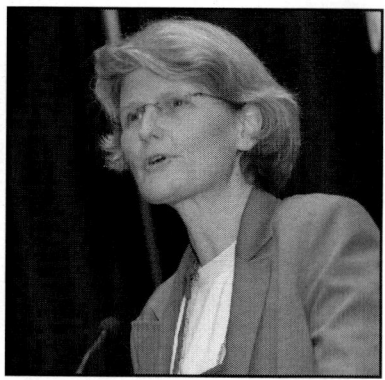

2018 William B. Graham Prize recipient Elizabeth H. Bradley at the 2008 Annual Meeting

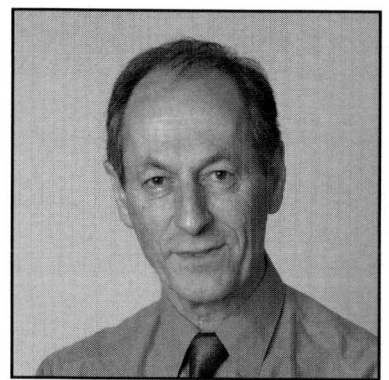

2008 William B. Graham Prize recipient Sir Michael G. Marmot

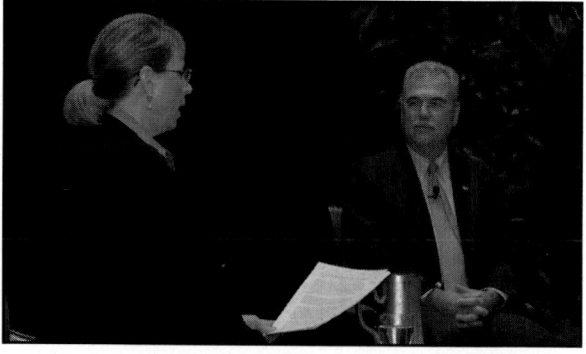

Former American Hospital Association President Richard Umbdenstock with then Board Chair Sharon Buchbinder, RN, PhD

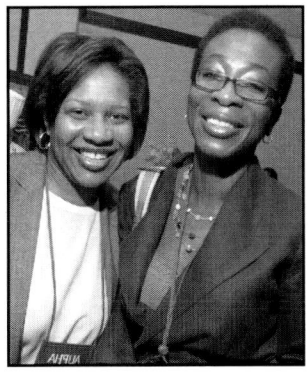

Members Carla Sampson, PhD, and Simone Cummings, PhD

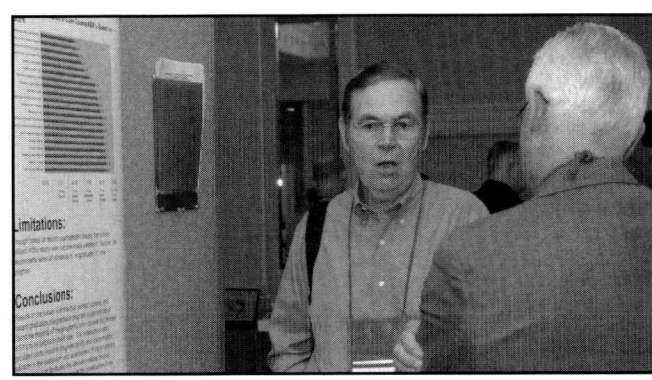

Member Myron D. Fottler at a 2008 Annual Meeting poster session

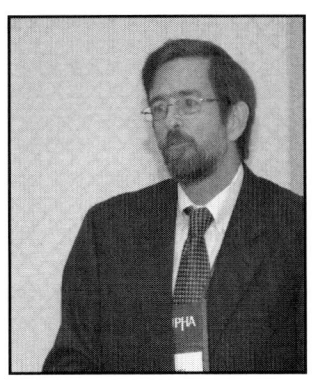

Current President and CEO Gerald L. Glandon, PhD, presenting at the 2008 Annual Meeting

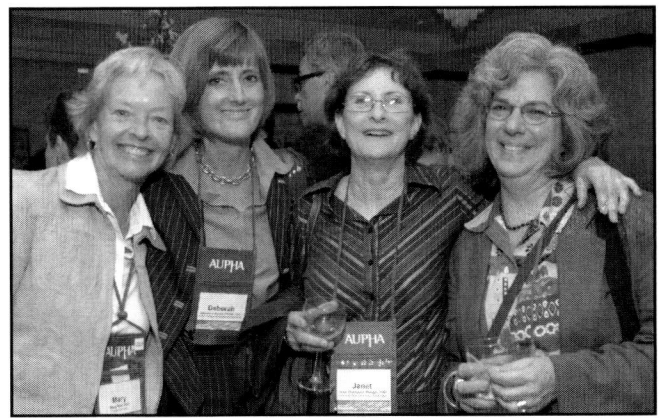

Past Chair Mary E. Stefl, PhD, current ACHE President Deborah J. Bowen, CAE, FACHE, Past Chair Janet Reagan, PhD, and member/former staff member Sherril Gelmon, DrPH

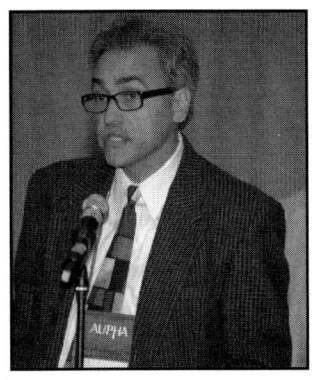

Louis Rubino, PhD, has questions for a speaker

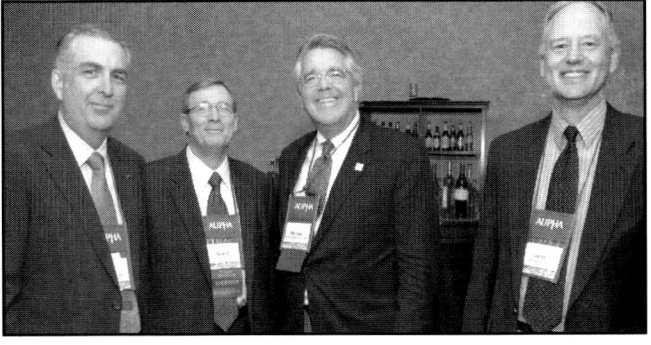

Members Eric Ford, PhD, Former Chair Grant Savage, PhD, Michael R. Meacham, JD, MPH, and John Huppertz, PhD, at the 2008 Annual Meeting

AUPHA 60TH ANNIVERSARY AT THE 2008 ANNUAL MEETING IN CHICAGO *(continued)*

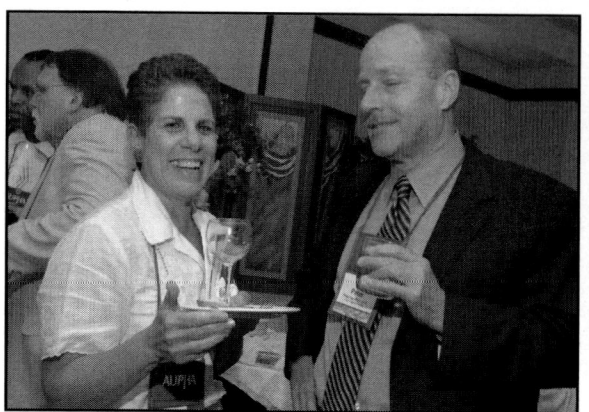

Current Board Member Carol Molinari, PhD, with former Board Chair Peter Fitzpatrick, PhD

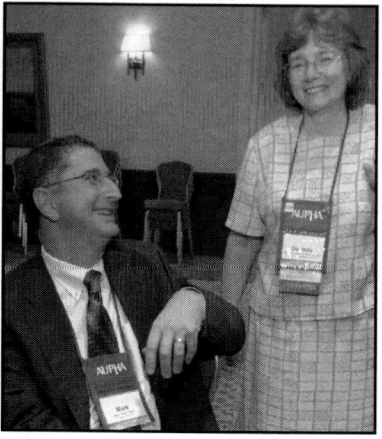

Current Chair-Elect Mark Diana, PhD, with member Dolores Clement, PhD

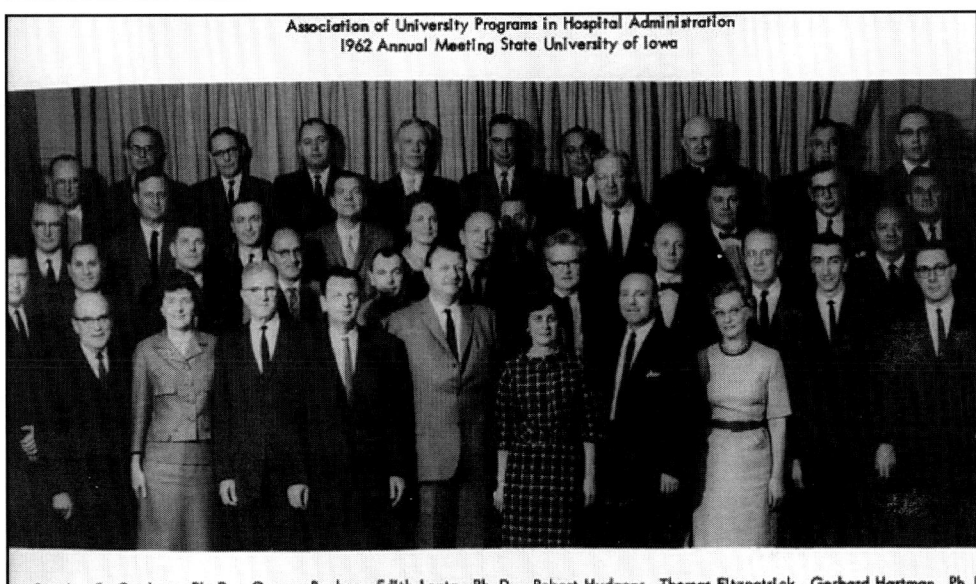

Association of University Programs in Hospital Administration
1962 Annual Meeting State University of Iowa

Row I   E. G. Jaco, Ph.D., George Bugbee, Edith Lentz, Ph.D., Robert Hudgens, Thomas Fitzpatrick, Gerhard Hartman, Ph.
        Ruth Inghram, Cecil Sheps, M.D., Eugenie Stuart, Lawrence Hill, Douglas Brown

Row II Walter Wentz, Col. Sam Edwards, Keith Taylor, Richard Durbin, John Thompson, Odin Anderson, Ph.D., Donald Smith
        Dean Conley, Antonio Vargas, M.D., Jose Gutiérrez, M.D., Leon Gintzig, Ph.D.

Row III Donald Caseley, M.D., Charles Frenzel, Samuel Levey, Ph.D., Andrew Pattullo, Sophie Zimmerman, Paul Lembcke, N
        Charles Cardwell, Donald Horsh, Frederic LeRocker, Cdr. Harold Civiello

Row IV Clement Clay, M.D., Elwood Camp, Charles Berry, Thomas McCarthy, Ph.D., Madison Brown, M.D., James Stephan,
        James Martin, Rev. John J. Flanagan, S. J., Cdr. Paul Austin, Floyd Patrick, Ph.D., Hilda Kroeger, M.D.

1962 Annual Meeting at the State University of Iowa

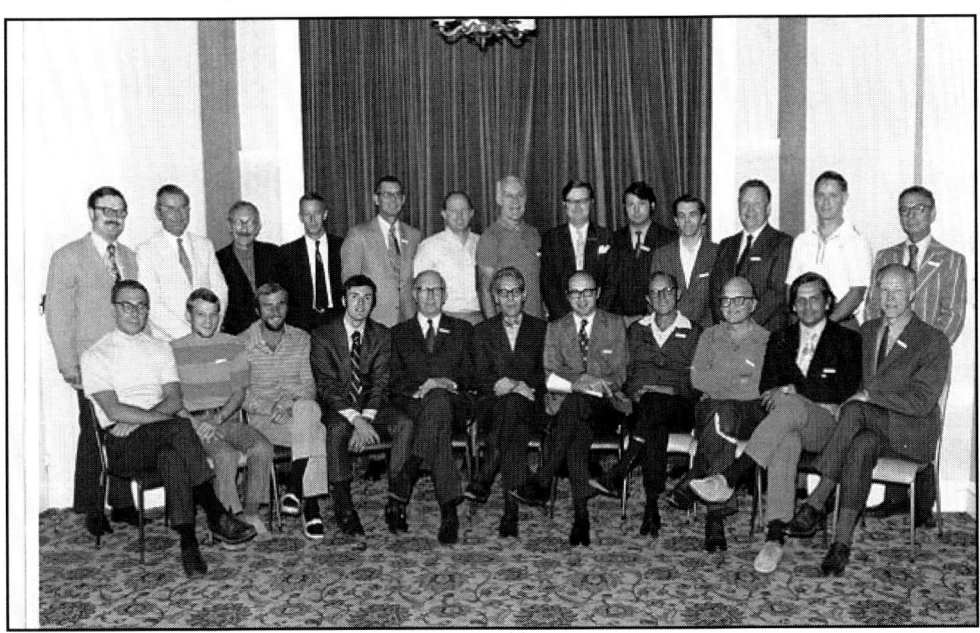

Members at an early meeting

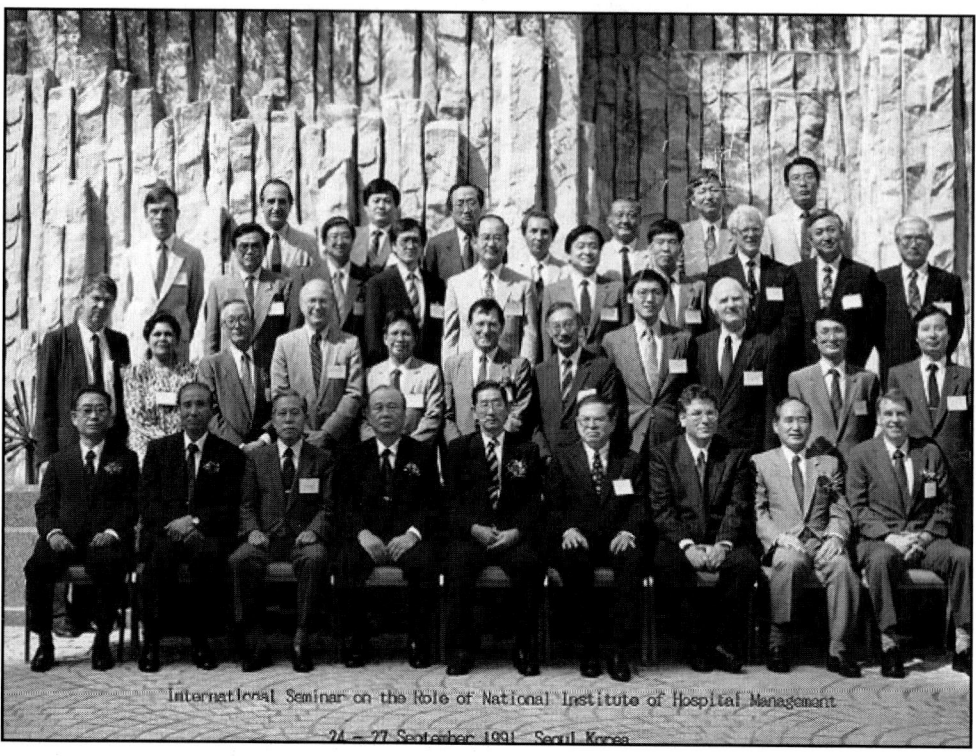

International seminar in Seoul, South Korea

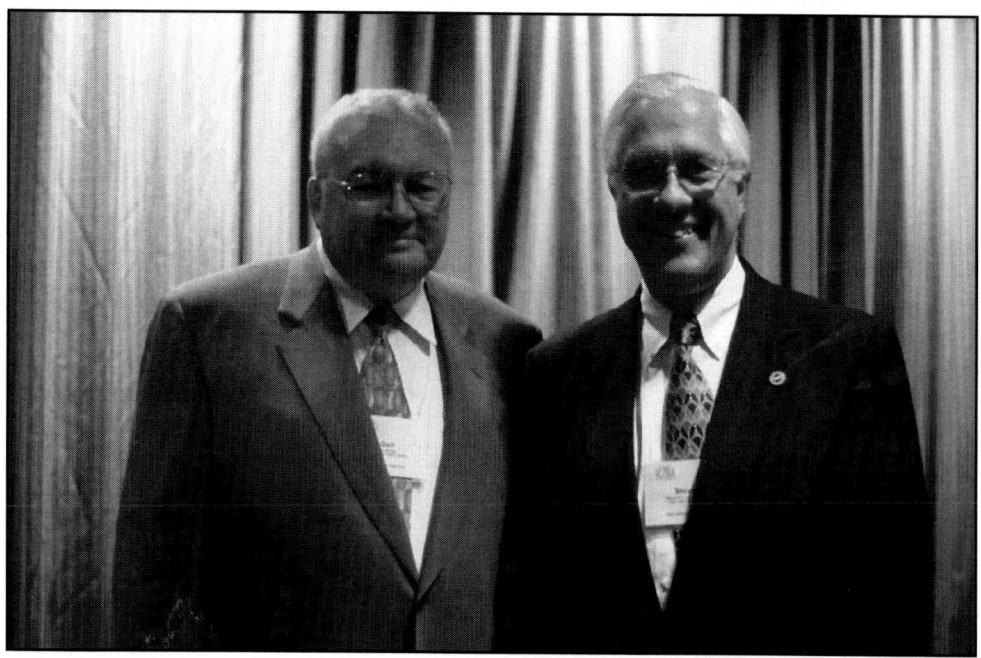

Gail Warden and Past Board Chair Steve Loebs, PhD

OTHER AUPHA PHOTOS *(continued)*

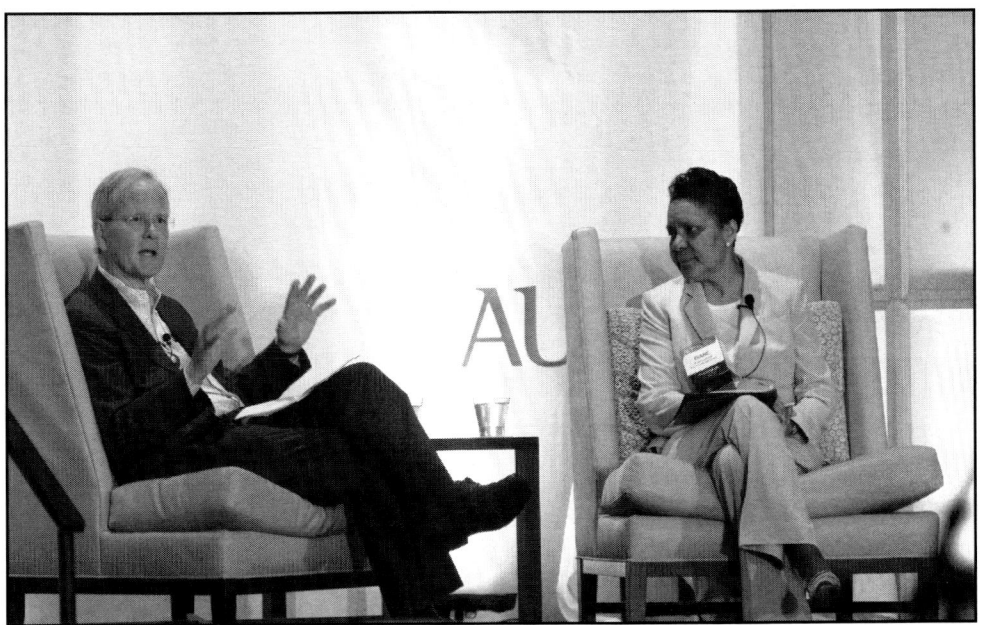

2016 Forum Speaker John Glaser with then Board Chair Diane M. Howard, PhD

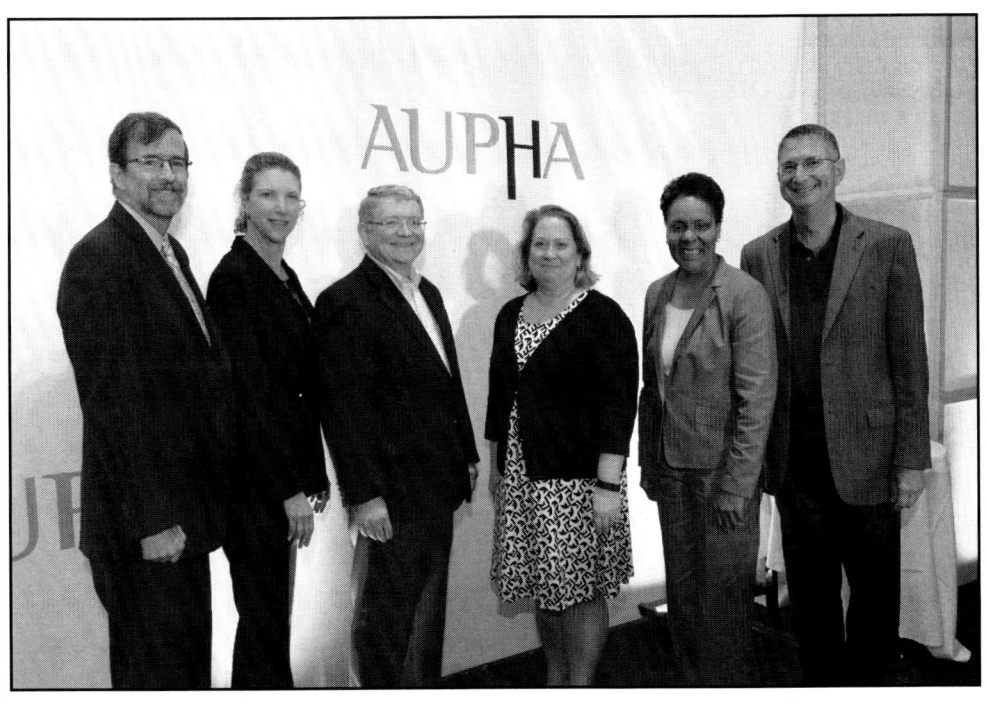

Members of the 2015–2016 Executive Committee

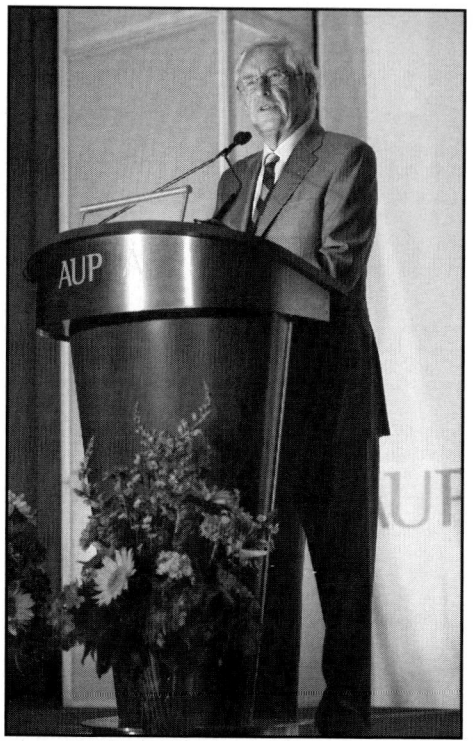

2016 William B. Graham recipient
John K. Iglehart

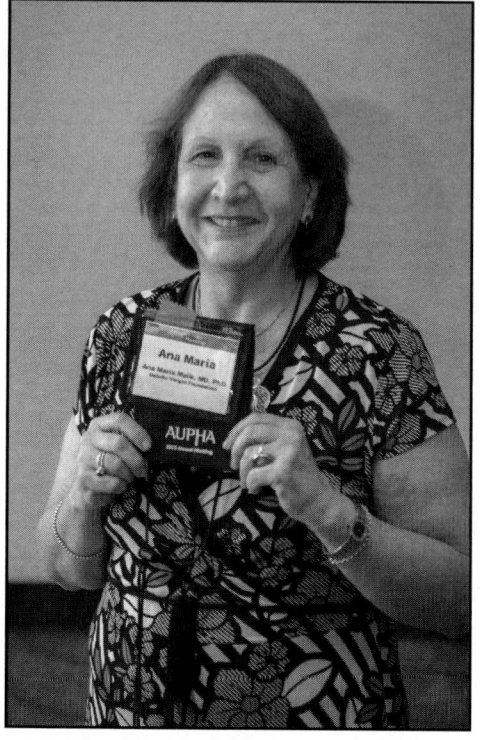

Member Ana Maria Malik, PhD, MD, at
the 2017 Annual Meeting

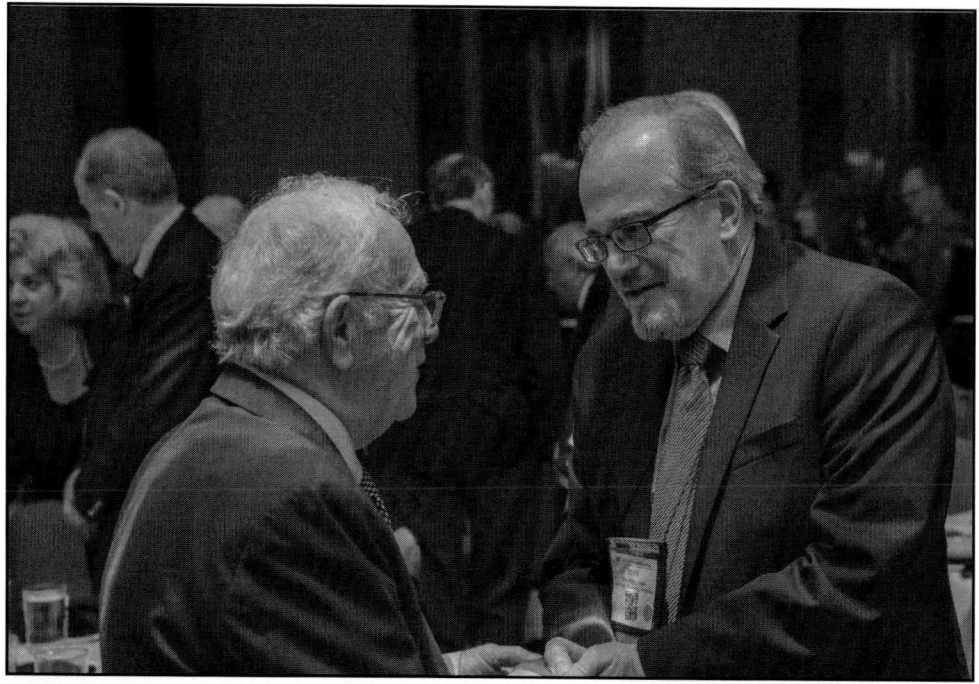

Brian Malec, PhD, with 2014 William B. Graham Prize Recipient Stuart Altman, PhD

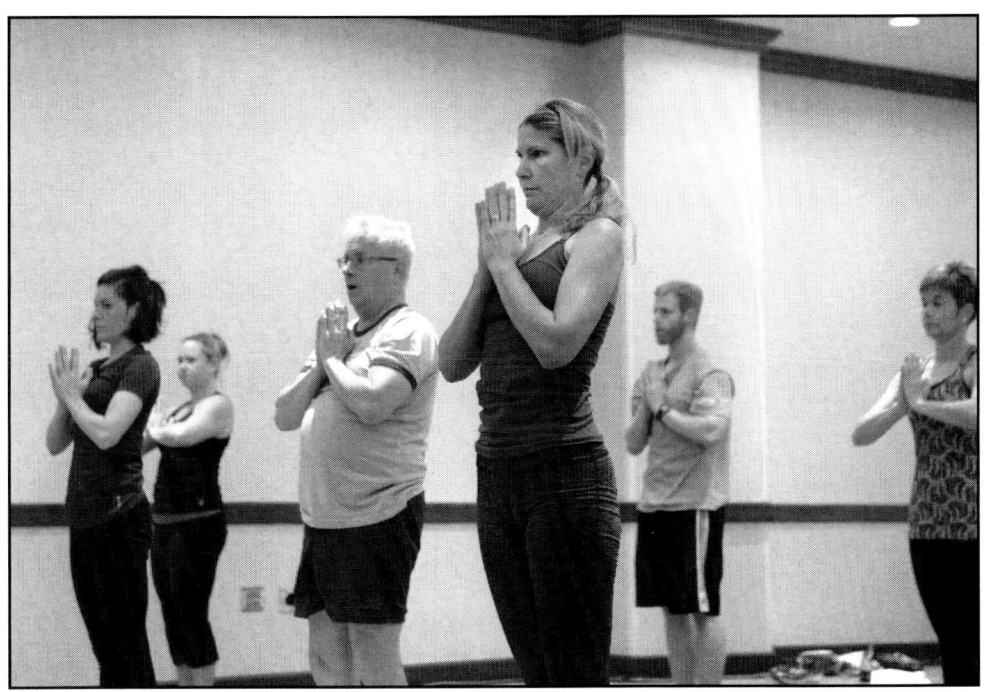

Conference attendees enjoying yoga at the 2017 Annual Meeting

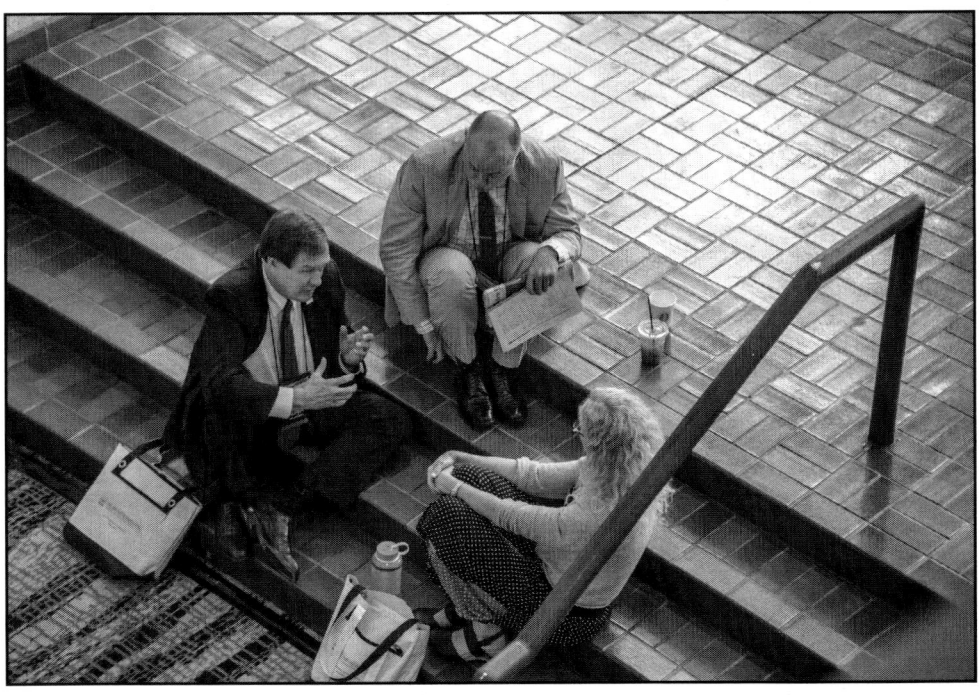

Brooke Hollis, PhD, Julie Carmalt, PhD, and Dan Gentry, PhD, taking a break at the
2017 Annual Meeting

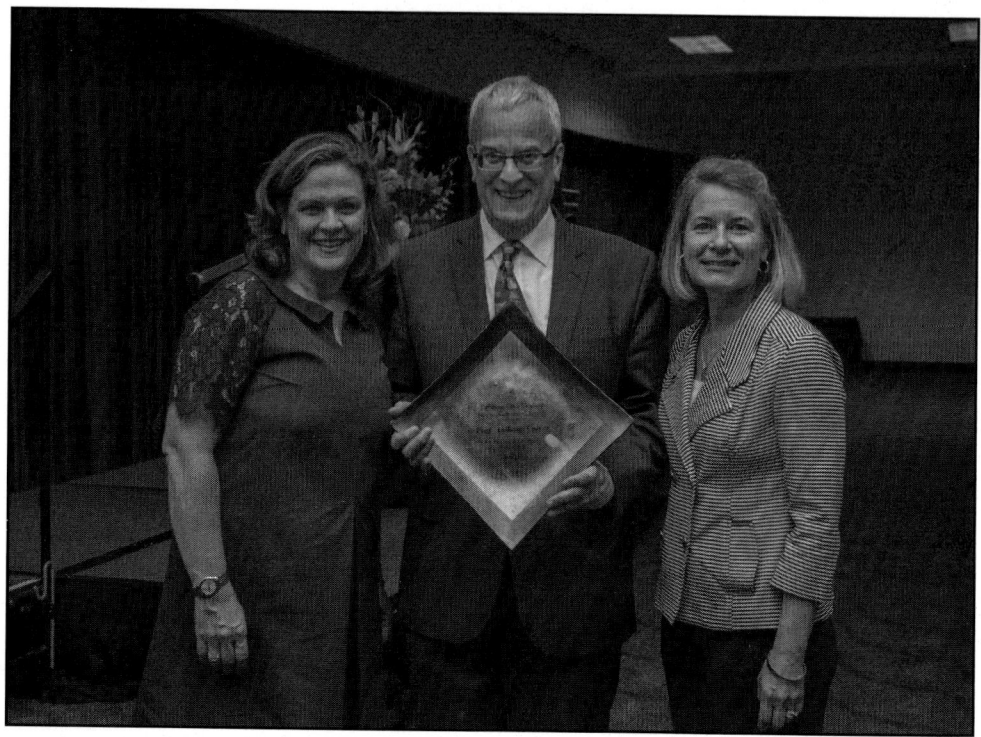

Tony Culyer, CBE, BA, Hon DEcon, Hon FRCP, FRSA, FMedSci, one of the 2015 Graham Prize recipients, accepts the award from Alice J. Campbell and Laureen M. Cassidy with the Baxter International Foundation

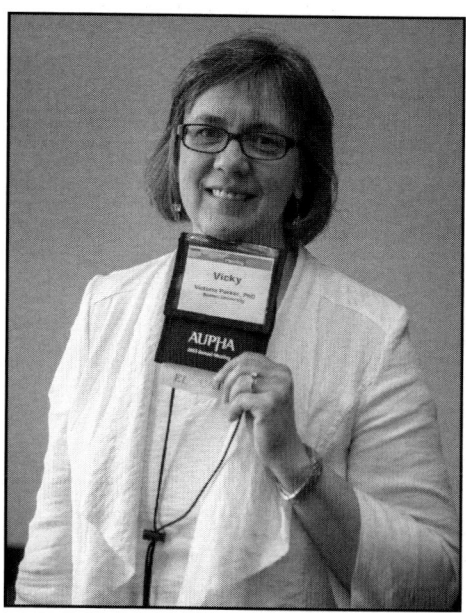

Member Vicky Parker, PhD, at the 2017 Annual Meeting

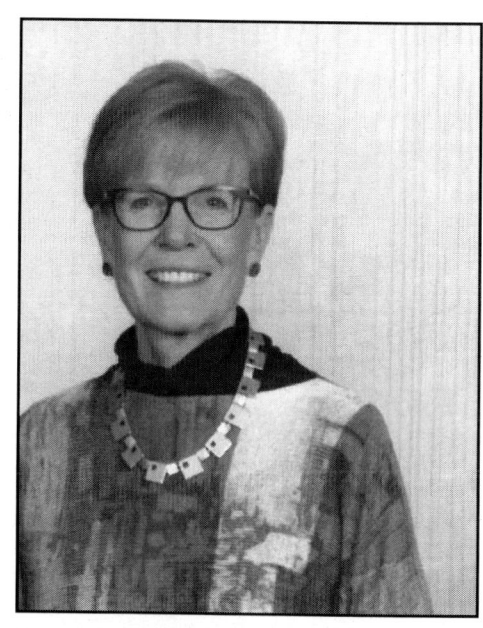

Former CAHME President and CEO Margaret Schulte, DBA